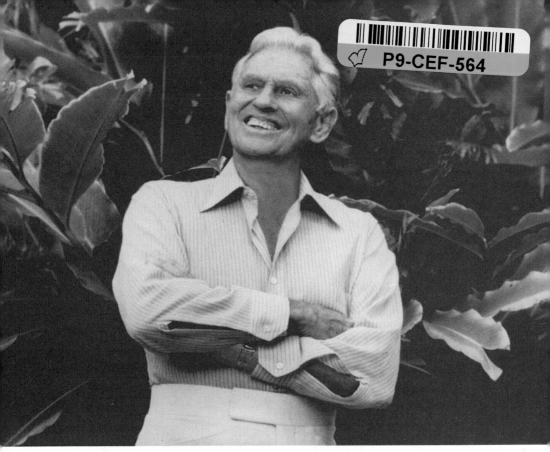

PAUL C. BRAGG, N.D., Ph.D.
World's Leading Healthy Lifestyle Authority

Paul C. Bragg's daughter Patricia and their wonderful, healthy members of the Bragg *Longer Life, Health and Happiness Club* exercise daily on the beautiful Fort DeRussy lawn, at world famous Waikiki Beach in Honolulu, Hawaii. Membership is free and open to everyone who wishes to attend any morning – Monday through Saturday, from 9 to 10:30 am – for Bragg Super Power Breathing and Health and Fitness Exercises. On Saturday there are often health lectures on how to live a long, healthy life! The group averages 75 to 125 per day, depending on the season. From December to March it can go up to 200. Its dedicated leaders have been carrying on the class for over 28 years. Thousands have visited the club from around the world and carried the Bragg Health and Fitness Crusade to friends and relatives back home. When you visit Honolulu, Hawaii, Patricia invites you and your friends to join her and the club for wholesome, healthy fellowship. She also recommends you visit the outer Hawaiian Islands (Kauai, Hawaii, Maui, Molokai) for a fulfilling, healthy vacation.

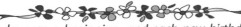

Your first birthday was a beginning, and each new birthday is a chance to begin again, to start over, to take a new grip on life. – Paul C. Bragg

Our Favorite Quotes We Share with You . . .
where space allows. We all need inspiring, informative words of wisdom to help guide us in our daily living.

Here's a wise ancient Turkish saying: No matter how far you've gone down on a wrong road, turn back and get on the right road!

Man is composed of such elements as vital breath, deeds, thoughts and the senses. – The Upanishads

I cannot overstate the importance of the habit of quiet meditation and prayer for more health of body, mind and spirit. – Patricia Bragg

Breathing is the movement of spirit within the body; and working with breathing is a form of spiritual practice. – Andrew Weil, M.D.

Dream big, think big, but enjoy the small miracles of everyday life.

When you live A Healthy Lifestyle *you can help activate your own powerful internal defense arsenal and maintain it at top efficiency. However, bad or sloppy breathing habits make it harder for your body to fight off illness.*

Every year I live I am more convinced that the waste of life lies in the love we have not given, the powers we have not used. – Mary Cholomondeley

When health is absent, wisdom cannot reveal itself, art cannot become manifest, strength cannot be exerted. Wealth is useless, and reason is powerless. – Herophiles, 300 B.C.

If you truly love Nature, you will find Beauty everywhere. – Van Gogh

God will not change the condition of men, until they change what is in themselves. – Koran

The natural healing force within us is the greatest force in getting well. – Hippocrates, Father of Medicine

When you live The Bragg Healthy Lifestyle you can help activate your own powerful internal defense arsenal and maintain it at top efficiency. However, if you continue unhealthy eating habits, it is harder for your body to fight off illness! – Paul C. Bragg

Stretch for health. Watch a cat stretch. Cats are graceful and coordinated. They instinctively stretch to keep muscles tuned and joints flexible. Notice how cats feel the stretch, test the tension, relax and focus on the stretch.
Order the famous book – Stretching – Call (800) 333-1307
by Bob Anderson, *World Famous Stretching Coach* – www.stretching.com
Breathing exercise illustrations in this book are by Jean Anderson.

ii

BRAGG
HEALTHY
LIFESTYLE
Vital Living to 120

Your days shall be 120 years.
Genesis 6:3

Formerly Titled:

TOXICLESS DIET,
BODY PURIFICATION
& HEALING SYSTEM

PAUL C. BRAGG, N.D., Ph.D.
LIFE EXTENSION SPECIALIST

and

PATRICIA BRAGG, N.D., Ph.D.
HEALTH & FITNESS EXPERT

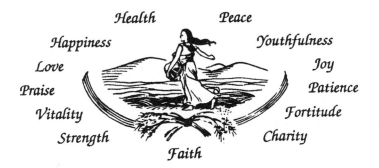

Health   *Peace*
Happiness   *Youthfulness*
Love   *Joy*
Praise   *Patience*
Vitality   *Fortitude*
Strength   *Charity*
Faith

JOIN
Bragg Health Crusades for a 100% Healthy World for All!

HEALTH SCIENCE
Box 7, Santa Barbara, California 93102 USA

World Wide Web: www.bragg.com

Notice: Our writings are to help guide you to live a healthy lifestyle and prevent health problems. If you suspect you have a medical problem, please seek alternative health professionals to help you make the healthiest informed choices. Diabetics should fast only under a health professional's supervision! If hypoglycemic, add spirulina or barley green powder to liquids when fasting.

BRAGG
HEALTHY
LIFESTYLE
Vital Living to 120

Formerly Titled: Toxicless Diet
Body Purifdication & Healing System

PAUL C. BRAGG, N.D., Ph.D.
LIFE EXTENSION SPECIALIST

and

PATRICIA BRAGG, N.D., Ph.D.
HEALTH & FITNESS EXPERT

Health Science, Box 7, Santa Barbara, California, 93102
Telephone (805) 968-1020, FAX (805) 968-1001
E-mail: bragg@bragg.com

To see Bragg Books and products on-line, visit our World Wide Web Site at: www.bragg.com

Quantity Purchases: Companies, Professional Groups, Churches, Clubs, Fundraisers etc. Please contact our Special Sales Department.

♻ This book is printed on recycled, acid-free paper.

- UPDATED AND EXPANDED -
Copyright © Health Science

Thirty-first printing MCMXCIX
ISBN: 0-87790-002-7

Published in the United States
HEALTH SCIENCE, Box 7, Santa Barbara, California 93102 USA

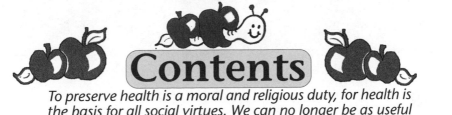

Contents

To preserve health is a moral and religious duty, for health is the basis for all social virtues. We can no longer be as useful when not well. – Dr. Samuel Johnson, Father of Dictionaries

Title

Remember: "It is NEVER too late to be what you might have been!"

When you sell a man a book you don't just sell him paper, ink and glue, you sell him a whole new life! There's heaven and earth in a real book. The real purpose of books is to trap the mind into its own thinking. – Christopher Morley

If I were to name the three most precious resources of life, I would say books, friends and nature; and the greatest of these , at least the most consistent and always at hand is nature. – John Burroughs

Laughter is inner jogging, good for your body and soul. – Norman Cousins

Living in harmony with the universe is living totally alive, full of vitality, health, joy, power, love, and abundance on every level. – Shakti Gawain

Contents

*Open thou mine eyes, that I may behold wondrous
things out of they law.* – Psalms 119:18

*We can no more afford to spend major time on minor things,
than we can to spend minor time on major things!* – Jim Rohn

*There is no biological reason why human beings should not reach
the age of 150.* – Dr. Alexis Carrel, The Rockefeller Institute

v

Contents

*When health is absent, wisdom cannot reveal itself, art
cannot manifest, strength cannot fight, wealth becomes
useless and intelligence cannot be applied.* – Herophilus

*Kindness should be a frame of mind in which we are alert to every chance:
to do, to give, to share and to cheer.* – Patricia Bragg

Bragg Healthy Lifestyle Vital Living to 120

Bragg Toxicless Diet, Body Purification and Healing System

This Course of Life Instruction is for those who want to learn how to improve, maintain and extend their health and live to a healthy 120 years! Millions worldwide have benefited and achieved Super Health from the message spread by my father and me. Now it's your turn to get started with The Bragg Healthy Lifestyle!

We are Pioneers in Health Crusading and love sharing with you – our readers and health friends! Soon after you start, the benefits from our health teachings will become amazingly apparent in your life and you will begin enjoying all of their wonder-working miracles!

This mind-opening, life-changing book helps you find and draw upon your body's own natural resources of health, energy and youthfulness! It teaches you to free yourself from the health wreckers that are destroying your health! It shows you how to flush out the toxins that cause most health problems. It also helps you eliminate stress, strain, tension and fatigue. Best of all, it helps you develop sparkling new supplies of health, zest and energy for a long, happy and fulfilled life!

The Bible promises us 120 years and with faith and strict observance of God's Eternal Health Laws we can make His promise good! "The Lord helps those who help themselves!" There is no reason why after reading this book, with your new understanding of how to live The Bragg Healthy Lifestyle, that you can't live a longer, healthier life even up to 120 years!

Your days shall be 120 years. – Genesis 6:3

Friends are the flowers in the garden of life.

The Toxicless Diet, Body Purification And Healing System Fully Explained

First, we want it definitely understood that this system does not claim to cure disease. No system can "cure" disease. No person can "cure" you of your ailments, aches and pains. Only the internal functions of your own body banish disease! The human body is self-cleansing, self-repairing and self-healing! You break a bone, the doctor sets the bone and puts it into a cast. The broken bone knits together again. After a certain number of weeks, the bone is again as strong as it was before the break – sometimes even stronger! There is no special diet, no special foods, no pill, no injection or prescription that can "cure" or mend a broken bone. The internal healing forces are within every human body – these are what heal and renew the bone!

Only Mother Nature Cures!

Burn this into your consciousness: Only Mother Nature Cures! Every human body has a special built-in healing mechanism. You cut your hand and three to five stitches might be required to close the wound. The doctor cleans, stitches and then bandages the wound. He can do no more. Now the miraculous healing mechanism of your body starts mending the wound.

Man's body was created according to the laws of physics and chemistry, which are the Creator's own laws. They never vary. His law is written upon every nerve, every muscle, every faculty, which has been entrusted to us. – Henry W. Vollmer, M.D.

The preservation of health is a duty. Few seem conscious that there is such a thing as physical morality. – Herbert Spencer

*A healthy body is a guest-chamber for the soul;
a sick body is a prison.* – Francis Bacon

The human body has one ability not possessed by any machine – the body has the ability to repair itself. – George W. Crile

The World Health Organization reported recently that 24.5 million people worldwide – nearly 50% of the yearly deaths – are victims of just 3 chronic conditions linked to unhealthy lifestyles : circulatory diseases (especially heart attacks and strokes), cancer and lung disease! – US News and World Report

Discover & Guard Your Body's Vital Force

To simplify this explanation of the Toxicless Diet, Body Purification and Healing System, we are going to call this vital healing power "Vital Force"! All of us must have this Vital Force energy in order to stay alive! When the Vital Force is completely exhausted, then there is death. Many people live at a very low rate of "physical vibration" because they have a very low amount of Vital Force. Then there are people who live a healthy lifestyle every day who enjoy a high rate of physical vibration with high energy! Their Vital Force is high!

Every day of your life you meet people with a high amount of Vital Force. On the other hand, every day you also see tired, exhausted, nervous, frustrated people full of aches, pains, diseases, stresses, strains and tensions. Most of these people are prematurely old . . . they appear and act older than their calendar years! People with a low quota of Vital Force have a low resistance to infectious diseases . . . they are the people who have frequent colds, flu, strep throat and many other disorders! They are the people who are chronically tired, suffering from what is often called chronic fatigue syndrome or Epstein-Barr. They are the people with poor memories who are full of aches and pains. They are lifeless, pale and often anemic. They are often unhappy, irritable people that nothing and no one can please!

Lack of Vital Force Brings on Enervation!

With the Vital Force energy at a low ebb enervation takes over. When enervation takes over physical troubles start to multiply! Remember first and foremost, we are miraculous instruments. In order for our bodies to be "in tune" and operate efficiently, there must be an adequate amount of Vital Force. It's needed to keep

the eliminative organs removing the accumulating toxins and wastes from our bodies daily. A clean internal body operates more efficiently, happier and better.

Deep breathing increases healing currents of Nerve Force and sends it throughout the body. – Patricia Bragg

There you have it – the secret of life in a nutshell! The body accumulates a certain amount of toxic waste from the food you eat. As the food passes through the gastrointestinal tract, the great intelligence of the body selects the nutrients it needs and the waste or residue is passed on and out of the body. This squeeze and push function requires a large amount of Vital Force. If a person has low Vital Force, food wastes don't pass out of the body in the normal time, then toxins build up.

The body has a warm temperature of 98.6 degrees. If food wastes remain too long in the gastrointestinal tract, daily toxic poisons build up. Then auto-intoxication and putrefaction starts to set in. Toxic poisons are then thrown back into the bloodstream and you start to self-poison and self-pollute! The many dangerous effects of this toxic poison being thrown back into the bloodstream can become devastating and deadly!

Enervation & Disease: Cause & Effect

Mother Nature always gives warnings when toxic poisons start to build up in the bloodstream – such as headaches. Some ache, others throb and then there are the worst of all, the severe migraine headaches. There are also many other symptoms of auto-intoxication – biliousness, nausea, mental depression, irritability, stress, tension and strain. The full list of symptoms is too long to enumerate here. Enervation slows down the eliminative functions not only of the bowels, but also the kidneys, skin and lungs. Our bodies cannot efficiently eliminate the accumulating toxic wastes when our Vital Force is in a sluggish, low vibration, enervated condition!

For every effect there must be a cause! All disease conditions are effects of enervation. The basic cause of enervation is a poor diet and an unhealthy lifestyle. The average food of civilization has been so perverted and robbed of its life and energy that most of its vital nutrients have been removed! You cannot expect to build a high Vital Force on poor fuel. Most humans in civilization suffer from chronic malnutrition. The prefix "mal" means ill or bad. So malnutrition means ill nutrition and in plain words adds up to bad health!

Thy Food Will Be Thy Remedy! – Hippocrates

On the Chios Island (now Khios) in classical Greece 2,500 years ago, Hippocrates, the bearded physician-teacher – father of medicine, sat in the shade of an Oriental plane-tree on a beautiful hillside. There Hippocrates taught and enlightened his medical students with these brilliant, factual, precise and ageless important words of wisdom.

Your Food Will Be Your Remedy . . . No one, to date, has more eloquently described a healthy way of life! The entire Toxicless Diet, Body Purification and Healing System is based on this one vital truth. This System is based on the principle that with healthy foods and fasting you can cleanse, purify and rebuild your body and find perfect health again. Yes, food can be your medicine!

My father, over the course of his entire, long lifetime, proved that within fruits and vegetables are the amazing natural remedies for most of man's physical problems.

The medical profession insists that it strives to emulate the Father of all physicians. Indeed, it requires its practitioners to take the Hippocratic Oath, one of the most sublime declarations of lofty ethics ever written. Yet today there are thousands of dedicated bacteriologists, pharmaceutical researchers and chemists sitting in gleaming laboratories throughout the world, busily turning out synthetic, so-called "magic" drug panaceas for every human misery. Unlike the wise Hippocrates, their unwise battle cry appears to be: "Thy remedy shall be our newly invented wonder drug."

The three greatest letters in the English alphabet are N-O-W. There is no time like the present. Begin Now! – Sir Walter Scott, Scottish Poet, 18th C.

There is only one corner of the universe that you can be certain of improving and that's your own self. – Aldous Huxley

The natural healing force within us is the greatest force in getting well. – Hippocrates, Father of Medicine

*The law, "**Whatsoever a man sows that he shall also reap**," is inscribed in flaming letters upon the portal of Eternity, and none can deny it, none can cheat it and none can escape it.* – James Allen

"Fast Relief" Claims Misguide Americans

TV, movies and videos are schools of wrong living, promoting fast foods and fast remedies, as well as crime, killing and lowering our morals and family principles! We must all protest! This unhealthy and unwholesome philosophy is promoting the downfall of America's health and family principles! Look at the TV commercials – the old and new remedies flash on the screen. We have all heard claims of, "Fast relief for headaches," with this remedy or the other. "Fast relief for acid stomach, heartburn and indigestion." "If your joints and muscles hurt, take this fast, fast remedy." Not only TV, but also radio, newspapers and magazines are full of remedies for all kinds of human physical and mental ailments.

Unhappy, anxiety-ridden people follow the warning voices of TV drug commercials that cost millions. They are made to believe that they can purchase health and energy at the drugstore in bottles filled with miracle powders, liquids or pills. They forgot or didn't know that health can be found only by obeying Mother Nature's healthy lifestyle laws.

6

Ailing, sickly people today are constantly looking for an instant "cure-all," some miracle substance that will restore their lost health and youth! The Toxicless Diet, Body Purification and Healing System is the intelligent way to follow the clear-cut laws of Mother Nature.

Foods Can Make or Break Your Health!

People are so steeped in their health-breaking habits of eating that they think some mysterious potion will do away with all of their physical miseries! They want to circumvent all their bad eating habits. They don't even realize that food can either make you a physical wreck or it can give you Health Supreme!

You are what you eat, drink, breathe, think and do. – Patricia Bragg

The destiny of countries depends on the way they feed themselves. – Brillat-Savarin

While whole grain products are an excellent source of magnesium – a vital element for maintaining healthy bone structure . . . studies have found that over 80% of magnesium is lost in the refining of grains into white flour!

Unhealthy "Dirty" Blood Causes Illness and Premature Ageing

Most humans will not face the realities of life . . . they live in a dream world. When you tell the average sick person that all their physical troubles are due to a "dirty, filthy bloodstream," caused by an unhealthy diet and lifestyle . . . often they are sensitive and insulted. They want all the modern tests and a specific diagnosis. Then the dear ones want a special name and special treatment given to their physical trouble or troubles. But they still want to smoke, drink alcoholic beverages, tea, coffee, soft and cola drinks and continue eating lifeless, demineralized, devitaminized, refined, bleached, dead foods filled with harmful, lifeless calories! They want their doctor to instantly banish their aches and pains! How can their physical troubles vanish when the individual keeps breaking important health laws?

There are No Miracle Cures Except Those Performed by Mother Nature and God!

This brings us to the Great Law of Compensation. You cannot get something for nothing! The precious health we teach and write about is a Super-High Health that you must earn by living a healthy lifestyle! No one can cure you . . . NO ONE CAN BANISH YOUR AILMENTS! Health works with this great Law of Compensation. Health building requires individual discipline! Your mind and brain must take over the operation of your precious body, because flesh is dumb! You can put anything into your mouth and swallow it. Only a clear, intelligent and reasoning mind will carefully supervise what is put in the stomach. Always remember that what you eat and drink today will be walking and talking tomorrow. Food is your fuel! Good healthy food makes fuel that gives good performance!

Studies show both beta-carotene and vitamin C, abundantly found in fruits and vegetables, play vital roles in preventing heart disease and cancers.

He who has health has hope; and he who has hope, has everything.
– Arabian proverb

Do You Show Signs of PREMATURE AGEING?

Is everything you do a big effort?
•
Have you started to lose your skin tone?
Muscle tone?
•
Do small things irritate you?
Are you forgetful? Confused?
•
Have voices begun to fade?
•
Has your vision started to dim?
•
Do you wobble a little when you walk?
•
Do you get out of breath
when you climb stairs?
•
How limber is your back?
•
Do your joints creak?
•
How well do you adjust to cold and heat?
•
Ask yourself this important question:
Do I seem to be slipping and
not quite like myself anymore?
If the answer to this question is "Yes,"
You had better do something about it!

START TODAY
Living The
Bragg Healthy
Lifestyle!

He who understands nature walks with God. – Edgar Cayce

You Become What You Eat

Because the human body is the most powerful miracle instrument, it can take years and years of the cruelest punishment from an unhealthy lifestyle. Then comes the day of reckoning when the body reaches its capacity for being loaded down with unhealthy grease, salt, sugar, preserved, refined and junk fast foods that produce a sick, clogged bloodstream! Then disease strikes with all its powerful force! Cataracts blind and blur the vision. Arthritis cripples and stiffens joints. Ears go deaf. Varicose veins cripple the legs. Ulcers form in the stomach and intestines. Piles and deadly fissures attack the rectum. These are just a few of over 4,000 crippling diseases that can make life a living hell while on this Earth!

These tragic things do not just happen . . . it's again the Eternal Law of Compensation at work. Disease is not like a thief in the night that creeps up on you and attacks you. You created the horrible condition which can often torment your every waking hour! These people who have, through ignorance or willfulness, brought themselves to this wretched physical condition, will cry out in pain and anguish, "Save me! Help me from my suffering and torment!" We are sorry to inform them that there is no simpler, more effective treatment to restore health and peace of mind than the cure Mother Nature provides through natural living.

Mother Nature is a hard taskmaster . . . disobey her laws and she will give you punishment that is almost beyond human comprehension. Go to any hospital and see the poor, wretched, suffering humans writhing on their beds of pain. These are the people who never learned the great natural laws. Many of them scoffed when well-meaning relatives and friends suggested that they live a healthier lifestyle. They were not going to give up their fun . . . so they smoked, drank alcohol, tea, coffee, cola and soft drinks and loaded up on refined

Use your willpower and better judgement to select and eat only foods best for you, regardless of ridicule from friends or acquaintances. – Dr. R. T. Field

Open your mind, for the doors of wisdom are never shut. – Ben Franklin

and dead foods to their hearts' content. If you tried to correct their ways, they had all kinds of excuses and answers to cover up their dietetic sins. "I am healthy," they would boast. "My grandmother lived to be 89 and smoked, drank and ate what she liked. I will be like my old grandmother!" But it did not work out that way. Now on their hospital beds they are helpless, broken humans ready for the human scrap heap.

Health Road or Sickness Road?
Which Road Will You Take?

Your health and the length of time you are going to remain on this earth are strictly up to *you* and *you* alone! You must make your choice! You can decide to travel the average (unhealthy) road. But seldom will someone tell you the errors of this way. No one will stop you! You will have lots of company. The average person takes their health and youthfulness for granted. They want the big thrills of life, or what they think are the big thrills . . . they do not have a correct sense of real values. "Live it up!" is their cry. "Eat what agrees with you and makes you happy," they say.

Again let us give you a serious warning . . . remember that you are going to pay dearly for every sin you commit against your body! The wages of sin are physical suffering and often early death!

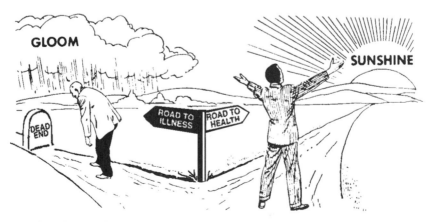

The choice of which road to take is up to the individual. He alone can decide whether he wants to reach a dead end or live a healthy lifestyle for a long, healthy, happy, active life. – Paul C. Bragg

Don't Clog the Pipes of Your Body

Our body is really a great plumbing system. We are made up of small pipes, medium-sized pipes and large pipes like the gastrointestinal tract, which is 30 feet long. Through the gastrointestinal pipe, from the mouth to the rectum, flow the food and drink we consume.

There is a great miracle muscular system within the gastrointestinal tract that propels the food slowly down and outward. To keep this muscular action efficient, the food we eat must contain bulk, moisture and lubrication. This is supplied by coarse raw vegetables such as cabbage, carrots, beets, celery, turnips, radishes and tender, young squash. All raw vegetables contribute to strengthen the muscular action along the gastrointestinal tract. We call raw vegetables and raw fruits "Nature's Broom." They are absolutely necessary if you are going to enjoy Higher Health and longevity! Even the American Cancer Society and the United States Surgeon General agree: eating fruits and vegetables is important for the prevention of cancer.

In our opinion, every disease – no matter what its scientific name – is basically caused by the clogging of the human pipe system! Any localized symptom is therefore merely the result of an extraordinary local clogging by the accumulated toxic poisons at that particular point. Any part of the pipe system can become clogged. The #1 killer of them all in America is "Heart Disease," the accumulation of matter (cholesterol, fats, toxins) that clogs the cardiovascular system and the heart!

One of the world's most deadly diseases is hardening of the arteries. The vicious toxic material that hardens the arteries can completely block them so that your life-giving, oxygenated blood cannot pass through. Hardening of the arteries does not happen overnight; it takes a long time to develop this fatal condition! Yet, authoritative sources claim that some people start to get hardening of the arteries at a very early age.

Everything in excess is opposed by nature. – Hippocrates, Father of Medicine

Coronary heart disease is due to a lack of oxygen to the heart.
– Dr. Dean Ornish, *Stress, Diet and Your Heart* • Web: ornish.com

Learn to Apply Health Lessons from History

Premature hardening of the arteries was observed even as early as the Korean War, when 350 soldiers were closely examined after death. These were young men, between the ages of 18 and 28. The autopsies revealed that every one of them had a certain amount of hardening in their arteries! There is little doubt that these young men had, since childhood, been fed on the typical unhealthy American diet. They ate meals high in fats, meats, cereals, desserts and other highly processed foods. Their devitalized, highly refined diet was heavily loaded with salt, saturated fats and refined white sugar. (Currently today it's *aspartame*, a toxic sugar substitute. See page 42 and the website: aspartamekills.com) Many doctors and studies agree that refined white sugar, salt and saturated fats lead to heart conditions and hardening of the arteries.

12

All of their lives these young men had been fed on commercially hardened fats of all kinds. They had all eaten smoked and brine-cured meats such as bacon, ham, sausage, luncheon meats and all the other kinds of preserved meats. They were also heavy users of processed, fast foods containing table salt (a harmful inorganic sodium) and preservatives. Table salt contains no organic minerals, vitamins, enzymes or nutrients. The naturally occurring organic sodium found in foods is the best source!

Why Does Premature Ageing Happen?

In other words, these young soldiers grew up on a diet of hardened fats, cholesterol and toxin-producing foods. As a result of their unhealthy diet they started to develop cardiovascular degenerative disease before the age of 30! Remember, clogging of the human pipe system can start when a youngster! This is the reason why many people prematurely age! It's sad that people age way before their time. In our world travels we find many people who look and act 20 to 30 years older than their chronological age! Why? It's their unhealthy lifestyles!

There are only two ways to live your life. One is as though nothing is a miracle. The other is as though everything is a miracle. – Albert Einstein

Forget Calendar Years – Be Ageless!

Study the people who are close to you. Look at their posture, walk and eyes – do you see good health and high energy or poor health and little energy? Look at their foreheads and temples and see how many veins pop out like small snakes. Many are quite deaf, many have poor vision and many have slow reflexes . . . they move stiffly and slowly and their brains think slowly. They become like the cemented living dead, a product of their unhealthy, harmful lifestyle of living!

These people may be in their 40s, 50s or 60s, but they are far older than their calendar years – prematurely old because of obstructions and clogging in their internal pipe systems. Their bodies are soaked and saturated with vicious, poisonous toxic materials!

Just because a person lives to be 60, 70, 80, 90 or more is no reason to believe that they should suffer from any degenerative disease such as hardening of the arteries. Most people's thinking is controlled by mob psychology. The average person has been trained to think falsely that as the years go by you are supposed to get older while deteriorating in body and mind. "Age brings on troubles" . . . that is what they have been told and that is exactly what they believe!

You cannot control your chronological years, but with The Bragg Healthy Lifestyle, you can most assuredly control your biological age . . . in fact you can almost hold it to a standstill! A healthy life is wonderful and fulfilling!

It's exciting to be active, healthy, alert and to be of help and of service to this world! My father and I love sharing with you – our readers – this great message of The Bragg Healthy Lifestyle in this book! Please open your mind, heart and soul and realize that you can be in control of your health and enjoy a healthy, long life!

Love makes the world go 'round, and it's everlasting when it's written with caring, loving advice that will improve and enrich your life! This is why my father and I love sharing with you the health wisdoms which can be with you on your long life's journey. Our books on health, fitness and longevity go 'round the world spreading health and love! – Patricia Bragg

Slow Me Down, Lord

Slow me down, Lord

Ease the pounding of my heart by the quieting of my mind.

Quiet my hurried pace with a vision of the eternal reach of time.

Give me, amid the confusion of the day, the calmness of the everlasting hills.

Break the tensions of my nerves and muscles with the soothing music of the singing streams that live in my memory. Help me to know the magical, restoring power of sleep.

Teach me the art of taking minute vacations or slowing down to look at a flower, to chat with a friend, to pat a dog, to read a few lines from a good book.

Slow me down Lord, and inspire me to send my roots deep into the soil of life's enduring values that I may grow toward the stars of my greater destiny.

"There is but one way to live and that is Mother Nature's and God's Healthy Way!"

Health comes about when the power which produces health is active and predominant; sickness is the result of the opposite power working in the opposite direction. – Plotinus, 2nd century A.D.

Always do what is right – despite any public opinions.

---

*If someone is going down the wrong road
he doesn't need motivations to speed him up.
What he needs is education to turn him around!*

Ponce de Leon,

Searched for the "Fountain of Youth."

*If he had only known
It's within us . . .
Created by the food we eat!
Food can break or make your health!*

Chapter 2

Steps to Agelessness And Longevity

Agelessness

We believe it is possible to live in a perfect state of agelessness. Let's reason it out together. Every 3 months you get an entirely new bloodstream, so it is not the bloodstream that gets old. Every 11 months, every cell in the body has renewed itself . . . so you have a practically new body every 11 months. Every 2 years you get an entirely new bone structure, so in 3 years you are really born again . . . the renewal process has taken place! Now, if you keep the body clean and purified by eating a diet that continually cleanses the body, how can you get sick? How can you get old? The only thing that can kill you is a disease or an accident. Time cannot kill you!

15

We have met in our many years of travel hundreds of people 100 and more years old; their eyes were perfect, they had no hardening of the arteries, no blindness, no aches and pains. Most of these people lived their early lives in rural settings where they never ate refined and processed foods. They lived active lives on simple, natural, healthy foods from their own surroundings.

If these people had known about The Bragg Healthy Lifestyle they could have controlled their life and the ageing process indefinitely and lived even longer!

Why Die Before Your Time?

Read in the Bible where some people lived 900 and more years in a state of ageless grace! Of course the skeptics will scoff at these ages and say, "They recorded time differently than we do." They will tell you it's impossible to live to be 900. But they have not studied

The more natural food you eat, the more you'll enjoy radiant health and be able to promote the higher life of love and brotherhood. – Patricia Bragg

these ancient people's habits. They lived on foods that did not obstruct and clog the pipe system. This was the only thing that kept them alive – a clean body, free from clogging, encumbrances and obstructions. And that is exactly what this Course of Instruction is going to give you – a clean, healthy body! The Bragg Healthy Lifestyle will help you keep the toxic poisons flushing out of the body. Who knows? You, our reader and new health friend, may live 100 years or more in abundant health by following The Bragg Healthy Lifestyle! We want this for all of you – a long, happy, healthy and fulfilling life!

Remember that death is brought to the body when it is so saturated and bogged down with toxic poison that it can no longer function to maintain life! Start now to be a good health captain of your entire life! Do not allow toxins into your body. Keep it clean and pure so that you will reap both super health and longevity!

The Garden of Eden

We believe man once lived in a tropical paradise. In all our research and study we have come to the definite conclusion that man once lived in a Garden of Eden, and his diet consisted of raw and cooked fruits and vegetables. We believe that the man of Eden ate many green leafy vegetables, and that he ate nuts and seeds. This is the diet we believe man lived on in Biblical times, with freedom from disease, and that some lived to be as old as 900 years or more.

Now we want to clarify this whole statement so we will not be misunderstood. We believe that man lived in this tropical paradise and that at no time did they have to worry about being cold. They could lie down at night and sleep without any discomfort or chill. This is the true state of man. But then we find this was to change because of the approach of the Ice Ages. All over the world lifestyles were altered many times by these climate changes. As man was forced to live in colder areas, the variety of fruits and vegetables available to him was naturally reduced and limited to seasonal crops.

Follow Mother Nature and God – the rewards are great! – Patricia Bragg

Vegetable Protein Percentage Chart

LEGUMES	%
Soybean Sprouts	54
Mungbean Sprouts	3
Soybean Curd (tofu)	43
Soy flour	35
Soybeans	35
Soy Sauce	33
Broad Beans	32
Lentils	29
Split Peas	28
Kidney Beans	26
Navy Beans	26
Lima Beans	26
Garbanzo Beans	23

VEGETABLES	%
Spinach	49
New Zealand Spinach	47
Watercress	46
Kale	45
Broccoli	45
Brussels Sprouts	44
Turnip Greens	43
Collards	43
Cauliflower	40
Mustard Greens	39
Mushrooms	38
Chinese Cabbage	34
Parsley	34
Lettuce	34
Green Peas	30
Zucchini	28
Green Beans	26
Cucumbers	24
Dandelion Greens	24
Green Pepper	22
Artichokes	22
Cabbage	22
Celery	21
Eggplant	21
Tomatoes	18
Onions	16
Beets	15
Pumpkin	12
Potatoes	11
Yams	8
Sweet Potatoes	6

GRAINS	%
Wheat Germ	31
Rye	20
Wheat, hard red	17
Wild rice	16
Buckwheat	15
Oatmeal	15
Millet	12
Barley	11
Brown Rice	8

FRUITS	%
Lemons	16
Honeydew Melon	10
Cantaloupe	9
Strawberry	8
Orange	8
Blackberry	8
Cherry	8
Apricot	8
Grape	8
Watermelon	8
Tangerine	7
Papaya	6
Peach	6
Pear	5
Banana	5
Grapefruit	5
Pineapple	3
Apple	1

NUTS AND SEEDS	%
Pumpkin Seeds	21
Sunflower Seeds	17
Walnuts, black	13
Sesame Seeds	13
Almonds	12
Cashews	12
Filberts	8

Data obtained from *Nutritive Value of American Foods in Common Units*, USDA Agriculture Handbook No. 456. Reprinted with author's permission, from *Diet for a New America* by John Robbins (Walpole, NH: Stillpoint Publishing).

17

Unhealthy Lifestyle and Heavy Proteins Shorten Life!

Now allow us to repeat this to make it clear in your mind. When man lived in his tropical paradise on a diet of natural, organically grown fruits and vegetables, he was constantly detoxifying and purifying his body. He lived every day on the Toxicless Diet, Body Purification and Healing System. Most lived a long life, free from aches and pains, diseases, premature ageing and senility.

When man left his paradise, the Garden of Eden, it necessitated his venturing into different climates. Then his diet was changed by necessity towards the eating of more grain foods like wheat, barley, oats, rye, maize and millet. He also learned to cultivate rice, lentils and beans of all varieties, which he dried and stored for long periods of time. Having his fruit and vegetable selection greatly reduced, he turned to the killing of animals for meat and the collecting of birds' eggs. In time he found he could domesticate animals like the cow, goat and fowl. Not only did these provide him with ready meat, but he also had a fresh egg supply, and it wasn't long before he mastered the milking of the cow, goat and the sheep.

From this milk he learned to make butter, cheese and other dairy products. So, from a predominantly healthy alkaline diet, climate changes forced man to slowly change his eating habits until his diet was one heavy in starch, proteins, fats and acids. Meat is very heavy in uric acid, which is quite toxic. Meat is mostly protein, but it also carries visible and invisible fats (the pipe-clogging waxy substance called cholesterol), along with any toxic waste, viruses, germs, chemicals, drugs, and the hormones, antibiotics and diseases that were in circulation in the animal's body at the time of slaughter.

Studies have revealed that fat stored in the body's "spare tire" around the waist increases the risk for diabetes, heart disease and shortens the lifespan!

Uninformed men, when pampered with meat and dairy products are much more choleric, mean and cruel in their tempers than those who live chiefly on fruits and vegetables. – William Smellie, 1780

The World is Our Human Classroom

As we travel the world, we study the eating habits of the people. Let us take the Eskimo who lives in the frigid Arctic on a diet of mostly animal and fish flesh and their blood. Their environment provides no other recourse but to rely on these foods. Results – they age prematurely and have a short life span. They are lucky if they reach 40! They suffer from stiff joints, bad livers and bad kidneys and many skin diseases.

Now, as we move down from the Arctic Circle into the countries like Lapland, Finland and the Northern European countries, we find people using lots of meat, fish, eggs and bread. We get a crystal-clear picture of what these foods do to these people. We see premature ageing in these countries, we see the loss of sight, hearing and the general deterioration of the body by the time people have reached 50. Many suffer from gum disease causing them to lose their teeth. Many have suffered their whole life with some nagging ailment, such as bronchitis, asthma, skin problems and other diseases.

Continue down into the tropics. Today you will find people who don't know how to eat the natural, Garden of Eden way! People in the tropics eat lots of pork, fowl, eggs, sugars, sugared drinks and white rice. Although they live in the tropics they have lost the natural instinct of living on the Toxicless Diet, Body Purification and Healing System! Now you see lots of disease and excess weight, plus leprosy, which is a dreadful disease.

People in the world's industrialized countries eat lots of meat; not only fresh meats, but all kinds of smoked, salted and preserved meats. Today people worldwide eat many products made with refined white sugar and now the sugar substitute – toxic aspartame (diet and soft drinks, candy, desserts, pastries, etc.), refined white flour (breads, doughnuts, pizza, etc.), white rice and processed cheeses, etc. There are over 2,800 chemical additives to color, preserve and stabilize refined, processed foods!

Men do not die, they kill themselves. – Seneca, Roman Philosopher

Widespread Use of Toxic Preservatives, Harmful Insecticides & Deadly Chemicals Is a Crime Against Our Health!

When they see their teeth and those of their children with cavities, people, in utter despair, start to put deadly fluorides in their drinking water, falsely believing that this will keep their teeth perfect and healthy. Read the Bragg book *Water – The Shocking Truth*. See back pages book list. Also read page 118. We want to share with you the importance of daily drinking 8 glasses of pure, distilled water – nature's great cleanser and purifier that helps operate all of your internal machinery!

And oh, what a sick, broken-down creature civilized man has become! He has Hospitals, Clinics, Doctors, Nurses, Bacteriologists, Pharmaceutical Researchers, Scientists and Chemists trying to do something to help him in his misery. In the United States, which is a representative country of these so-called civilized countries, 47 times every second a prescription is filled by a white-coated chemist at one of the over 100,000 pharmacies in the United States! The staggering cost of these many colored tablets, capsules and lozenges amounts to more than a shocking $30 billion a year!

CIVILIZED MAN IS SICK, has been for a long time, and is getting sicker! He has almost reached a point of total helplessness. Not only are the adults sick in body, but they are sick in mind. 30% of the hospital beds in our civilized countries are occupied by people suffering from some mental condition. Nearly 1 out of 10 children are now born either crippled or developmentally disabled. The insane asylums and mental wards of the civilized world are packed to overflowing. If the truth be told – there are many more thousands of extremely ill and mentally unstable people (some dangerous to themselves and others) who should be institutionalized as well! Civilized man has strayed from the humble Garden of Eden, where he lived enjoying long years of perfect health and happiness on natural purifying foods.

You Can Create Your Own Garden of Eden

My father and I want you to know we have no illusions that there is any place left in the world that could be called the 100% perfect Garden of Eden. But if you want to be well and live long, you must work to create your own Garden of Eden to the best of your ability wherever you live! You should strive to live in the most environmentally pure and safe surroundings as possible! Drink only distilled or reverse osmosis-purified water. Eat organic fruits and vegetables. Buy and use air purifiers for your home, office and even your car. This is what we do wherever we have lived. When possible we put in organic vegetable gardens, fruit trees and flowers to best create our own Garden of Eden!

That is exactly what the Bragg Healthy Lifestyle is going to do for you. It will help you establish – wherever you are – your own Garden of Eden! We cannot expect to have the health, vitality and long life that our brothers and sisters enjoyed in the original Garden of Eden. But we can, through careful control of our diet, purify our bodies by flushing out and eliminating altogether the vicious toxic poisons that are causing us illness, suffering and premature ageing.

Naturally there will be a lot of compromises to make. America has had many generations of eating an unbalanced and highly refined, unhealthy diet. It's important to begin the trip back to the Garden of Eden slowly, wisely and cautiously. You can do it – start now!

You can't beat Mother Nature. Proctor and Gamble's synthetic fat, Olestra promises our fat-laden public the taste we love without the calories. The FDA has approved its use, but thousands of consumers have already suffered so many forms of gastric distress that the manufacturer has placed a warning label on their packages. The Harvard School of Public Health found that the synthetic fat also blocks carotenoids. These have been found to be important in fighting heart disease, cancer, stroke, and macular degeneration. Dr. Walter C. Willett, a medical doctor and scientist assigned to study the synthetic fat stated "there will be no benefit from Olestra in terms of weight reduction".

The USDA has issued new dietary guidelines encouraging more exercise and the consumption of less fat. The guidelines also stress the use of dietary sources of vitamins and minerals, especially antioxidants and B vitamins, including folic acid. In addition, the guidelines point out that diet is important to health at all stages of life and helps reduce the risk of diseases of all kinds.

Step 1: Rid Yourself of Toxic Foods – Detox

The beginning of this program must start with your avoiding the foods and drinks that dangerously clog, obstruct and throw waste into the human pipe system, the organs of the body and the cells. Study the Foods to Avoid List on the next page. Play it safe and healthy – never again let these foods pass through your body!

They work slowly, but very effectively and quite fatally! The first 35 to 40 years of life most people can willfully or ignorantly attempt to break the laws of human biochemistry. Some people have stronger constitutions than others. People will often make the statement to us that "My Grandfather is 88 and smokes, drinks alcohol and eats any food he wants to, and he is still living!" We have to listen to this occasionally because there are the lucky few who inherit a body that has wide arteries and wide veins. They are born with a capacity to burn poisons three times faster than the average person! But just remember this: when a person who is now 88 years old was born, 86,000 others were also and he is the lone survivor. One out of 86,000 is not a very good percentage!

Now, on the other hand, if that man had known about the Toxicless Diet, Body Purification and Healing System and had kept toxic materials down to a minimum, he might have lived to be 150! We have met many men and women from 100 to 125 years of age.

So the first thing you must do is to discard forever the so-called foods and potentially harmful products listed on the next page that humans put into their bodies.

Step 2: Analyze Your Own Health

The next thing to do before you go on The Bragg Healthy Lifestyle is to sit down and carefully analyze yourself! You know how you feel. No one in the world could diagnose in detail your problems. Therefore you must do a little self-diagnosing. You have read the list of clogging and toxic-forming foods. Only you know within your own heart how many unhealthy, dietetic indiscretions you have made and over how many years.

Avoid These Processed, Refined, Harmful Foods

Once you realize the harm caused to your body by unhealthy refined, chemicalized, deficient foods, you'll want to eliminate these "killer" foods. Also avoid microwaved foods! Follow The Bragg Healthy Lifestyle to provide the basic, healthy nourishment to maintain wellness.

- Refined sugar , artificial sweeteners (aspartame) or their products such as jams, jellies, preserves, marmalades, yogurts, ice cream, sherbets, Jello, cake, candy, cookies, chewing gum, soft drinks, pies, pastries, tapioca puddings and all sugared fruit juices and fruits canned in sugar syrup. (**Health Stores have healthy, delicious replacements, so seek, buy and enjoy!**)

- White flour products such as white bread, wheat-white bread, enriched flours, rye bread that has white flour in it, dumplings, biscuits, buns, gravy, pasta, pancakes, waffles, soda crackers, pizza, ravioli, pies, pastries, cakes, cookies, prepared and commercial puddings and ready-mix bakery products. (**Health Stores have huge variety of 100% whole grain products, delicious breads, crackers, pastas, pizzas, desserts, etc.**)

- Salted foods, such as corn chips, potato chips, pretzels, crackers and nuts.

- Refined white rices and pearled barley. • Fried and greasy foods.

- Refined, sugared (also, aspartame), dry processed cereals – cornflakes etc.

- Foods that contain olestra, palm and cottonseed oil. These additives are not fit for human consumption and should be 100% avoided .

- Peanuts and peanut butter that contains hydrogenated, hardened oils and any mold that can cause allergies.

- Margarine – full of dangerous, unnatural, trans-fatty acids.

- Saturated fats and hydrogenated oils – enemies that clog the arteries.

- Coffee, decaffeinated coffee, China black tea and all alcoholic beverages. Also all caffeinated and sugared cola and soft drinks.

- Fresh pork and pork products. • Fried, fatty and greasy meats.

- Smoked meats, such as ham, bacon, sausage and smoked fish.

- Luncheon meats, hot dogs, salami, bologna, corned beef, pastrami and packaged meats containing dangerous sodium nitrate or nitrite.

- Dried fruits containing sulphur dioxide – a toxic preservative.

- Don't eat chickens or turkeys that have been injected with hormones or fed with commercial poultry feed containing any drugs or toxins.

- Canned soups - read labels for sugar, starch, flour and preservatives.

- Foods containing benzoate of soda, salt, sugar, cream of tartar and any additives, drugs, preservatives; irradiated and genetically grown foods.

- Day-old cooked vegetables, potatoes and pre-mixed, wilted salads.

- Pasteurized, filtered vinegars, distilled, white, malt and synthetic vinegars are the dead vinegars! (We use only our Bragg Organic Raw, Unfiltered Apple Cider Vinegar with the "mother" as used in olden times.)

23

So you balance your ailments against your diet – you may have had bronchitis or asthma for many, many years – all this must be taken into consideration before you can live completely on the Toxicless Diet, Body Purification and Healing System. You've got to consider if you have had any operations. You've got to consider how many harmful foods and drugs you have used. You then not only have to get the food toxins out of your system, but if you have used drugs of any kind, they too are buried deeply into the tissues and must be flushed out!

The next consideration is how far your vitality has been lowered, and just how much Vital Force still remains in your body. The various physical troubles you have had to date in your life, as well as any drugs you have taken, all must be taken into consideration. Ask yourself these vital questions: How much meat do you eat? How many eggs do you eat? How many dairy products do you eat? These questions will all have to be carefully considered. After all factors have been responsibly analyzed you are ready to move on to the third step in the program.

Step 3: Your Individual Transition Diet

We want you to remember first, and bear in mind at all times, that the ideal diet of man is raw and lightly cooked fruits; raw, steamed or baked vegetables, brown rice, beans, legumes, raw nuts and seeds. Include an abundance of raw and lightly cooked green-leafed vegetables, such as chard, spinach, beet tops, turnip greens, mustard greens, collards and kale. We do not expect you, unless you are very ambitious about a thorough internal cleansing, to try to reach the ideal state of purification. There are various degrees of health that can be obtained by controlling the diet. We feel that if a person can reach the point where their diet contains from 60% to 70% raw or lightly cooked fruits and vegetables – with a minimum amount of protein, fats and sugars – they can live in a higher state of health for many long and vigorous years.

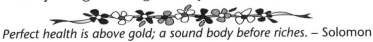

Perfect health is above gold; a sound body before riches. – Solomon

The Transition Diet starts first with a distilled water fast for 24 hours. (For some variety of liquids on fast days see page 100 - lower half.) Fasting is the greatest of all detoxifiers because, when we stop eating, all of our Vital Force which was used to masticate, digest and assimilate the food and eliminate the waste is used to purify the body! All this powerful energy is then used to release and to flush the accumulated obstructions and toxic poisons from the body! After each fast of 24 hours you must make it an iron-firm rule always to begin every meal with something raw. This will re-educate the 260 taste buds of your mouth to the delicate natural flavors of raw foods. Of course this cannot be accomplished if a person smokes cigarettes, cigars or a pipe, because taste and flavors are wasted completely on a smoker. The same goes for alcohol, tea, coffee, cola and soft drinks.

Please eliminate smoking, alcohol and all unhealthy beverages from your diet. Table salt (from both land and sea sources) must also be entirely eliminated on this cleansing diet. From this day on put no table salt (inorganic sodium) in or on your foods! Organic sodium occurs naturally in foods. Add delicious, healthier flavors to meals with herbs, onions, garlic, Bragg Liquid Aminos and Bragg Organic Apple Cider Vinegar! (See back pages for info.)

Step 4: Your Important Healing Crises

The healing crisis is one of the great mysteries of the Toxicless Diet, Body Purification and Healing System. Most humans have been so indoctrinated with the idea that when you have something wrong with you and you want to improve your health, you go and get a physical examination. You are then "diagnosed" and a name is given to your ailment. Treatment is begun and you believe that you are going to feel better, stronger and will soon "get well." Now don't expect to feel this way on the Toxicless Diet, Body Purification and Healing System! As you start on this System of Purification you are going to stir up old toxic poisons, and you do have plenty of them! Everyone else also has them, because almost everyone carries from 5 to 10 pounds of deeply buried toxic poisons in their bodies at all times. That is the reason it is so ridiculous when we hear people say, "I am healthy."

When they make that statement to us we say, "Let us put you on a fast – followed by the Toxicless Diet, Body Purification and Healing System – and we'll show you how much of these deeply buried poisons you have stored in your body."

That's what sickness is in the final analysis – the body becomes so corroded and loaded with vicious toxic poisons that it throws up its own cleansing purge or healing crisis. This healing crisis is the body's urgent response to the need to get clean and healthy! This cleansing can take the form of a cold, flu, pneumonia, fevers, headaches, coughs, earaches, boils, skin eruptions, abscesses and hundreds of other manifestations of the body ridding itself of toxic poisons. Disease is no mystery to us! These toxins do not come like a thief in the night, but are slowly created by an unhealthy diet and lifestyle habits, eventually leading to the accumulation of deadly toxins in the pipe system and every organ of the body.

26

So be ready for a series of cleansing and healing crises if you desire vitality supreme! This is a compensation action – this is your Vital Force asserting itself! You cannot get away from paying your price to Mother Nature. There is no way to circumvent this punishment for the crimes you have committed against your body! You must fast, cleanse, purify and heal your body.

We are not going to tell you that when you go on the Transition Diet – along with your 24 hour weekly fast, combined with eating more fruits and vegetables and eliminating some of the heavier foods – that you are going to feel good right away. You will not feel your best until you have eliminated a large amount of the hidden toxic poisons from your body.

We don't give special diets for special ailments. We don't believe in curative diets. We believe that you must slowly, through fasting and eating more raw organic fruits and vegetables, help your body flush out the heavy accumulation of toxic poisons that have built up over the years!

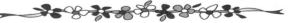

We live not upon what we eat, but upon what we digest. – Abernethy

What wound did ever heal but by gentle degrees. – William Shakespeare

Step 5: Reaping Health Benefits of Our Environment

Our bodies are fine instruments. The cleaner they become through the Toxicless Diet, Body Purification and Healing System, the more oxygen they will absorb, which is the source of all life. A toxin-polluted body can only take in so much oxygen when it is encumbered with so many obstructions! As you purify your body, it will feast on the invisible foods of the universe! Your body will absorb more oxygen, more energy, more ozone and more of the sun's strength-giving, gentle rays. Think of it – living on the invisible foods of Mother Nature! Babies do this – they eat only a small amount of food, and mother's milk is only 3.5% protein. Have you ever watched a healthy, active baby kick and wiggle and coo for hours at a time? Where is the energy coming from? Not from the mother's milk with only 3.5% protein! That baby's body is so clean that it has gathered from the universe the powerful, invisible nutrients. Look at the baby's delicate skin, look at his wide, bright eyes, at his sunny smile and listen to his powerful lungs support his cries when he wants something or he's wet!

Now look at the average person of 75 and notice their wrinkled, lifeless-looking flesh! Their eyes may be covered with cataracts and their eyelids drooping, making them look almost like human caricatures. Don't tell us it is because they are 75 and the baby is only a few months old! The difference is that the old man has been soaking up toxic poisons for most of his life. He is most likely suffering from toxemia – the clogging of his human pipes and organs as a result of a lifelong intake of unhealthy, toxin-forming foods.

Experts in healing feel that illness, especially after an emotionally cataclysmic event such as the death of someone close or a divorce, is one way the body expresses energy that's not being directed towards true desires and needs. Getting in touch with that which is truly important is not always that easy. Ways to overcome this problem and "reset" your life include keeping a journal, exploring your unexamined self through group therapy, prayer, listening to quiet music, taking life one hour at a time, and learning to love and improve your physical body and tell yourself how great you are! Life is a series of moments that you can take care of – make the most of them. – New Woman

Feed Your Pets as Well as You Do Yourself!

A man at 75 really might have only lived half of his lifetime! We support this statement with the fact that most animals live from 5 to 7 times their rate of maturity. Years ago we had an older pet dog that was about to go into heat. Determined that she would bear the healthiest litter possible, we fed her an extra super-balanced nutritional diet, supplemented with vitamins. There was only one pup born and we called him "Vitamin." He was an exceptionally healthy and beautiful pup. We kept him that way throughout his 154 years of life by feeding him only the most nutritious foods.

Our buddy and friend "Vitamin" enjoyed eating almost everything we ate: beans, rice, lentils, potatoes, carrots and other vegetables – these we mixed with his healthily-prepared dog food. We also sprinkled his food with big flakes of brewer's yeast (nutritious in B-complex vitamins, boron, etc.) to enhance his health and help keep fleas away. He liked his water "spiked" with a dash of our Bragg Organic Raw Apple Cider Vinegar which helped keep his body germ-free! ACV also helped keep his body limber and free from the stiffness of arthritis.

28

Most dogs and cats enjoy small slices of raw beef heart and chewing on large, raw bones and so did "Vitamin." To this day, all our dogs and cats live a healthy life, free of disease and health problems. Yes, our "Vitamin" did live to be 154 years of age since, relative to human years, a dog's and cat's year is equivalent to 7 years lived by a human. He actually lived 22 long years, and even at this age he was still quite an active, healthy dog. Sadly, he died in his twenty-second year after an accident.

Step 6: The "No Breakfast" Program

Our combined experience of over 140 years has proven to us that a carefully selected and progressively changed Transition Diet is the best way for every person to obtain their fulfilling goal of Total Health. But when people still live on unhealthy, refined foods, they must

---

Fasting is the greatest remedy – the physician within! – Paracelsus, *15th century physician who established role of chemistry in medicine.*

not eat too many fresh fruits and vegetables at first. Also every person must learn, if they truly want to attain perfection, they should not eat a heavy morning breakfast that saps their energy! See Pep Drink, page 114.

You will continually hear people say, "Breakfast is the most important meal of the day." This is simply not true! Scientifically, it takes a tremendous amount of nervous energy to chew, digest, absorb and eliminate a typical American breakfast. The average person believes that a hearty breakfast is going to give them strength. They believe this having been brainwashed by commercials and propaganda created for the producers of modern breakfast products: cereals, breads, pancakes, waffles, eggs, sausage, bacon, tea, coffee, cocoa, milk, etc. It is in their financial interest to have people believing they need a big breakfast for lots of energy.

Toxic Wastes and Poisons are Killers!

If we could only burn into your consciousness the one simple fact that toxic poisons and wastes are the agents that deteriorate and slowly kill human flesh, we'd feel that half of our work is accomplished! Naturally an adult that lives an active life in the sun and the fresh air is going to have a more mature skin than a 5-month-old baby, but that doesn't mean it must appear to be an old skin! We have seen men and women in their 80s, 90s and older who barely had a wrinkle or line on their face. Dr. John Harvey Kellogg was one of the greatest American health doctors who ever lived. The last time my father saw him, the famous doctor was giving a health lecture in his ninety-third year! He had the skin of a young man and a smooth face that literally shined with health like a polished apple! This is what my father and I wish for you, our new health friend and reader – a face and body glowing with super, optimum health!

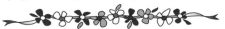

Wake up and say, "Today I am going to be happier, healthier and wiser in my daily living as I am the captain of my life and am going to steer it for 100% healthy lifestyle living!" Fact: Happy people look younger, live longer, happier and have fewer health problems! – Patricia Bragg

Progress is impossible without change, and those who cannot change their minds, cannot change anything. – George Bernard Shaw

DON'T LET JOHNNY APPLESEED'S DREAM DIE!

*The legendary "Johnny Appleseed" (John Chapman) between 1800 and 1849 wandered the wilds of the Ohio Valley planting apple trees. Over 150 years later some of these trees are still bearing fruit. But in today's world large seed companies are striving to make what Johnny Appleseed did illegal. Giant companies like Monsanto, producer of the Terminator seeds (pages 42 & 104), are striving to stop farmers from saving and reusing their seeds from generation to generation. They require farmers to sign a licensing agreement which strongly prohibits the reuse of Monsanto seeds. They even hire investigators like the Pinkerton Detective Agency and have others spy on their neighbors to identify farmers who break their contracts. It's bad enough that they have turned America's heartland into a farming police-state – but it's absolutely unforgivable that they seek to keep third-world farmers (who usually cannot afford to buy new seeds every year) from feeding billions of people who depend on their crops. Johnny Appleseed, one of the great American heroes, dreamed of a land covered with blossoming apple trees, a land where no one would go hungry. Now, 150 years later Monsanto has replaced Johnny Appleseed's joyous dream with a new and evil one of profit and famine. **We must protest Monsanto and their efforts to control the world's seeds, plants and the people's food!** Write and alert your congressmen, senators, and talk to family and friends to make them aware! Learn more about this shocking situation, protest and spread the word! View web: sedos.org*

30

It is important for each of us to have a special private area for ourselves – a place set aside for daydreaming, reading, meditation and prayer to help us rejuvenate from everyday life! This area can include anything that is meaningful and inspiring, including music you like. It should be a special place in your home, garden, etc. where you go to relax and reconnect with your inner self – a secret garden where you can grow and be nurtured.
– UC Berkeley Wellness Newsletter

Nature's Wonder Working Phytochemicals Help Prevent Cancer

Make sure to get your daily dose of these naturally occurring, cancer fighting substances that are abundant in onions, garlic, beans, legumes, soybeans, cabbage, cauliflower, broccoli, citrus fruits, etc. The winner is tomatoes, which contain the largest amount of miracle phytochemicals! See chart on page 131.

The greatest tragedy that comes to man is the emotional depression, the dulling of the intellect and the loss of initiative that comes from nutritive failure. – Dr. James S. McLester, Former President A.M.A.

Happiness is the meaning and the purpose of life, the whole aim of human existence. – Aristotle

Chapter 3

Vitality From the Universe

People Who Refuse to Grow Old

Doctors' offices throughout the civilized world are filled with women who suffer from menstrual problems, PMS, etc. We must sadly note that 7 out of 10 women reaching 60 in the United States have had some type of major problem or surgery on their female organs!

In our professional work as Health and Fitness Advisors to the Film Stars of Hollywood, we have many female clients who absolutely defy time! They have reaped the benefits of the Bragg Healthy Lifestyle – the Toxicless Diet, Body Purification and Healing System. You can never quite determine their age because at 50 they look 30, while at 60 look and act like only 40! This is what we want for both women and men; to look, feel and act years younger and have a huge zest and go-power for a healthy, long life!

The outward signs of this age-defying youthfulness are a straight-backed and handsome posture, supple breast contours, healthy smooth skin on face and neck, firm muscles and that particular vigorous grace typical of an active, healthy female. At age 50, 60, 70, and more these women still look quite attractive and youthful.

To the emotionally mature woman, this physical attractiveness is rarely an end in itself; rather, it's a subtle, psychological means by which she relates to the world around her. This quality derives its charm from a woman's balanced physical and mental self-confidence.

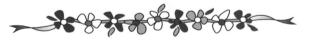

You don't get old from living a particular number of years; you get old because you have deserted your ideals. Years can wrinkle your skin, renouncing your ideals wrinkles your soul. Worry, doubt, fear and despair are the enemies which slowly bring us down and turn us to dust before we die. – Douglas MacArthur

Happiness is a rainbow in your heart, a real health sparkler! – Patricia Bragg

Ageless and Youthful – Why Not?

Now, thanks to The Bragg Toxicless Diet, Body Purification and Healing System, it is possible for women to retain their vitality – as well as their physical and sexual appeal – throughout their long, healthy life! By retaining these attributes, she also safeguards a less direct, more elusive aspect of her total feminine personality.

We believe that women can remain active, youthful, feminine, graceful and useful for their entire long life! Becoming old-looking can be a thing of the past for any woman who will invest the time and has the discipline to purify her body by living The Bragg Healthy Lifestyle!

Men, we're not forgetting you . . . this applies to you, too! We know that women typically take better care of themselves. Many men destroy themselves with tobacco, alcohol and a heavy meat, fat and sugar diet. It is a well-known fact that women live anywhere from 5 to 10 years longer than the average man! For most men a couple of beers and a pizza or a big steak and a large pile of fried potatoes is "good eating." That's one reason that men are dying off prematurely in alarming numbers! Our civilized world is full of widows simply because a large majority of men are ignorant about the importance of living a healthy lifestyle! They ridicule the very idea of good nutrition. They reject the value of eating fresh fruits, fresh juices, vegetables, salads, etc., as well as getting sufficient exercise to tune the body's machinery and muscular structure.

Most men are health sinners! Left to their own resources they will try to live on a bacon, sausage and eggs, strong coffee, biscuits and gravy diet and later a white flour pizza and beer diet. This is the reason our obituary columns are filled with death notices of men in their 60s, 50s, 40s and even some in their 30s!

Studies show repeatedly that exercise – particularly impact exercises like brisk walking, tennis, square dancing, cycling, aerobics and weight lifting – help you maintain a healthier body and build stronger bones!

The unexamined life is not worth living. It is time to re-evaluate your past as a guide to your future. – Socrates

If only these misguided souls had followed our health teachings, they could still be alive, enjoying a healthy, vibrant life and pizza, too! A tasty, satisfying and nutritious meal for everyone is a whole grain pizza topped with fresh pineapple, artichoke hearts, grated zucchini and carrot, chopped tomatoes, olives and lots of onion and garlic! Sprinkle with parmesan cheese and a spray of Bragg Amino Acids (delicious, all purpose seasoning, with 16 vital amino acids). For more recipes like this, read our *Bragg's Complete Gourmet Recipes,* which has 448 pages filled with hundreds of tasty, nutritious recipes that will enhance your life. See Bragg book list on back pages.

Not only do many men die young but, either through ignorance or willfulness, they will not follow the principles of natural nutrition and soon suffer from many physical ailments! The average man of 40 in most countries today is a candidate for a heart attack or some other chronic disease and an early death! Most men living on this heavy, meat-toxic diet lose their Adam Power very early in life! Our civilized world has men in their 30s – 40s complaining of being totally impotent! Many of these men suffer from a diseased, enlarged prostate.

33

Yet we have men in the TV and film industry who, through following our advice, have been able to retain their boyish figures. They also have youthful voices even though they are in their 50s, 60s, 70s and even more. They feel and act at least 20-30 years younger than their actual age! Also, we have consulted with top business men who are now in their 60s and 70s, yet look only 30 or 40! Why stop wanting to look younger? Start living The Bragg Healthy Lifestyle to look, feel and act years younger! Conrad Hilton did and got 20 more years! It's never too late to make healthy changes in your lifestyle!

I have the wisdom of my years and the youthfulness of The Bragg Healthy Lifestyle and I never act or feel my calendar years! I feel ageless! Then why shouldn't you? Start living this Bragg Healthy Way today! – Patricia Bragg

Laughter is inner jogging, and good for your body and soul. – Norman Cousins

Self discipline is your golden key; without it, you cannot be happy.
– Maxwell Maltz, M.D.

Conrad Hilton Thanks Bragg for His Long Life!

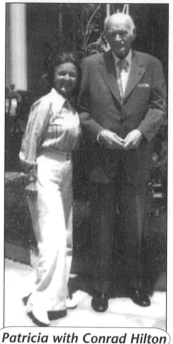

Patricia with Conrad Hilton

When the world's biggest hotel magnate Conrad Hilton was all of 80 and lying on his deathbed, we gave him a new lease on life by introducing him to The Bragg Healthy Lifestyle. He followed our instructions and discovered a whole new healthy, vibrant lifestyle! He was soon healthy, happy and fit, enjoying life! He even remarried at 88 years young! He remained active in business (half days at his office) to almost 100 years young! Mr. Hilton at 88 was quoted in a *People Magazine* interview as saying, "I wouldn't be alive today if it wasn't for the Braggs and their Bragg Healthy Lifestyle!" With this article was a photo of the grateful hotel millionaire with his healthy lifestyle teacher.

Eternally Youthful – Bob Cummings

Bob Cummings – one of Broadway and Hollywood's early successes of this century, also pioneered TV with his wholesome family series "My Little Margie". He carefully followed The Bragg Healthy Lifestyle for most of his long life from 18 when he was the toast of Broadway. Bob was the singing and dancing Star of Ziegfeld's Folly *"A Pretty Girl Is Like a Melody."* At his mother's insistence, Bob attended a Bragg Health Crusade lecture in New York City's Times Square on his one night a week off. It changed his life! My father's message penetrated Bob's heart, soul and mind, inspiring him to become a faithful Bragg follower. We are always proud to note that when Bob reached his 70s, he retained the youthful energy and posture of a man in his 30s!

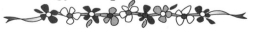

Man is fully responsible for his nature and his choices. – Jean Paul Sartre

Jack LaLanne Thanks Bragg for His Healthy, Successful, Long Life!

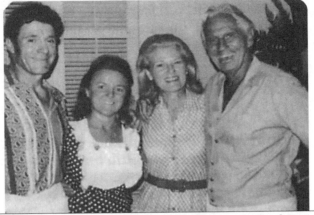

Jack LaLanne, Patricia, Elaine LaLanne & Paul Bragg

Jack says, "Bragg saved my life at age 15, when I attended the Bragg Health and Fitness Crusade in Oakland, California." From that day, Jack has continued to live The Bragg Healthy Lifestyle, inspiring millions to health and fitness!

Another success story and example of how attending one of our Bragg Health Crusade lectures can change someone's life with Total Health is found in a once-sickly 15 year old now famous for the 35 year run of his TV exercise show – Jack LaLanne! Over 69 years ago Jack's mother dragged her ailing son to a lecture being given by my health crusading father. They arrived late, the hall was packed, and they had to sit on the stage close to Dad in front of some 3,000 people. As Jack says:

I had dropped out of school for over a year. I was a shut-in! I had pimples and boils, and wore glasses. I was thin and so weak I had to wear a back brace and couldn't participate in sports. I didn't want anyone to see me.

I was weak and sick. I used to have blinding headaches every day and I couldn't stand the pain. I wanted to get out of this body I had. Paul Bragg told me I could be born again and be healthy, strong and fit if I changed to his healthy lifestyle.

He asked me, 'What do you eat for breakfast, lunch and dinner?' And I told him, 'Cakes, pies and ice cream!' He said, 'Jack, you are a walking garbage can.' That night I got down on my knees, by the side of my bed, and I prayed. I didn't say, 'God, make me a Mr. America.' I said, 'God, please give me the will-power and intestinal fortitude to refrain from eating unhealthy, lifeless foods when the urge comes over me. Please give me strength to exercise when I don't feel like it. God was good and inspired me to be strong and healthy!'

Jack LaLanne is Healthy, Youthful & Ageless

There hasn't been a jelly donut in his life since! LaLanne has faithfully followed The Bragg Healthy Lifestyle since that night. Jack now spreads the gospel of health and exercise through TV, lecture tours and by performing a series of extraordinary physical feats. This happily married father of two celebrated his 70th birthday with a mile-long swim . . . towing 70 rowboats carrying 70 people to show his super health and strength. Jack LaLanne is still going strong, healthy and youthful at over 84 years young and his body is like he's 30!

Toxic Poisons Cause Impotent Men, Frigid Women, Shattered Marriages and Families!

No wonder divorce rates of "civilized" countries are staggering. Impotent men and frigid women can't hold up the loving physical end of marital relationships! The majority of divorces in civilized countries are caused by physical incompatibility. When toxic poisons get into the reproductive glands of both male and female, serious problems arise! Sexual desires diminish as more toxic chemicals build up in the body's delicate organs.

There is no biological reason why men and women cannot retain their sexual energies up to 90 and longer! There is a great deal of proof in the world that this is true. One need only to look at the children that actors Charlie Chaplin and Tony Randall and artist Pablo Picasso fathered in their 70s and 80s for proof of the human machine's incredible, long-lasting fertility! In fact, a male's fertility can last an entire lifetime! The only thing that can happen to the reproductive organs of both

Health and love make everyday a honeymoon! – Patricia Bragg

Studies show that the average overweight American diets three times a year in an effort to lose excess weight, often going on expensive reducing programs, when all they have to follow is The Bragg Healthy Lifestyle!

the male and female is a diseased condition caused by an unfortunate incident, accident or the individual's ignorance of the importance of living a healthy lifestyle. Remember, we are punished by following bad habits of living, while we are rewarded for following good ones!

You Will Enjoy Internal Youthful Cosmetics and Long-Lasting Health

As you progressively eliminate the meat, sugars, fats and highly refined, processed foods from your diet and start eating more raw fruits, vegetables, salads, sprouts, fresh juices and whole grains, etc. you will soon begin to notice your skin and muscle tone improving. This starts your cleansing, healing and rejuvenation process! Also, try dry skin brushing and water therapy, pages 124-125. You are now on the road to eternal youthfulness! Remember, fresh fruits and vegetables are the internal cosmetics that reveal their wonder-working power by giving you healthy skin that glows like a fresh healthy, polished apple!

You have just begun to reap the many rewards of The Bragg Healthy Lifestyle! First you eliminate your body's obstructing toxic poisons. Soon your aches, pains and physical miseries will start to vanish! Then your energy is lifted to a higher degree and you no longer suffer from excessive fatigue. Yes, these changes will be life-changing and miraculous! Life is so precious and you will be proud for the improvements you are making in your life! You are taking responsibility for your own health and fitness as the captain of your life by steering towards super health, happiness and longevity!

Our creator would never have made such lovely days, and given us the deep hearts to enjoy them, unless we were meant to be immortal. – Nathaniel Hawthorne

Breathing is the greatest pleasure in life. – Papini

We are a product of our thoughts – and so is our health! While doctors and medicine have their place, self-healing is the most powerful medicine of all. Accepting the present and placing trust in a higher power frees your energy to focus on improving your life! See problems as challenges of growth, not as a punishment or judgment! Focus on happiness, forgiveness, hope and peace of mind, as well as physical change to ease any problems and situations.

You Can Create a New Healthier You!

When you faithfully follow The Bragg Toxicless Diet, Body Purification and Healing System, you will see some startling changes in the mirror. When you start the elimination process, occasionally you look wretched. This sometimes happens during the cleansing-healing crisis, when the greatest amount of toxic poisons are being flushed out of the pipes and vital organs of the body. After you have gone through several cleansing-healing crises you can then see the New, Healthier You revealing itself! Your eyes become brighter, your skin and muscle tone healthier and the joints of your body more supple. Your entire body throbs with a state of well-being that makes you glad to be alive!

Each day when you live on the Toxicless Diet, Body Purification and Healing System you make changes and adjustments that help create a new stronger, more vigorous and healthy body! To my father and I it's worth all the effort and dedication that goes into living this healthy lifestyle. Man has strayed from it because of the pressures of our modern, highly commercial world as we approach the 21st century. If he is to survive and live a healthy life, man must change over to a healthier lifestyle!

As we have stated, the degree of physical perfection you wish to attain is solely a personal matter and up to you! You must remember that 60% to 70% of your diet should consist of raw organic fruits, vegetables, sprouts and fresh juices. Your protein, plus your natural sugars, natural oils, natural starches and carbohydrates will make up the balance of your diet.

We must remind you that we offer no special diets for any specific ailments. We recognize only one cause for all ailments – internal toxic clogging! When you loosen and flush these vicious obstructions from your body, then you are taking The Bragg Royal Road to Total Health!

It's supposed to be a professional secret, but I'll tell you anyway. We doctors do nothing. We only help and encourage the doctor within. – Albert Schweitzer

To lengthen thy life, lessen thy meals. – Benjamin Franklin

It Takes Time and Dedication
To Reach Internal Perfection!

Constantly keep in mind that it took you years to get in the condition you are now, through an unhealthy lifestyle and bad dietary habits! Now you must be patient with yourself and Mother Nature and your body. Do not throw caution to the wind! If you have been eating meat several times daily, or eggs and cheese every day, you must slowly eliminate excessive use of these clogging foods. Soon your body won't even miss them!

As you continue to fast 1 day a week while adding more fresh, raw fruits and vegetables to your diet, you will gradually reach a perfect health balance! This is the point where toxic poisons are no longer retained in the body and it becomes mucus-free and toxin-free. This means you have reached a peak of internal fitness, a point of perfection! This is the condition everyone should seek! This is what we want for you, our new health friends and readers: to live a long, vibrant, healthy lifestyle and enjoy eating a healthy, balanced diet while maintaining a clean, painless, tireless and ageless body!

Caution – Move Slowly and Patiently
For Super Healthy Success in Your Life!

Keep in mind that "the wheels of time move slowly, but surely." You can't rush your body or Mother Nature! You can't be impatient and expect to reach perfect internal fitness in a few months! Rome wasn't built in a day! Achieving Super Health takes both dedication and time!

What You Eat – Becomes You!

Let's look at it from a cold, scientific viewpoint. If you eat a breakfast of hot or cold cereal or hot cakes with two eggs, bacon, three slices of buttered toast and some beverage like tea or coffee, it is not immediately converted into strength and energy! You must realize it takes a great deal of time and energy for your stomach

---

He who understands nature walks with God. – Edgar Cayce

Chew your liquids and chew your solids until they are liquid. – Paul C. Bragg

to mix this unnecessary, heavy breakfast with the digestive juices for the slow process of digestion and assimilation. Then the separation process takes place as the proteins are broken down by special juices in the stomach and the fats, starches and sugars are pushed into the small intestine for later digestion.

All foods need a large amount of special juices and enzymes to break them down so that they can be sent into the bloodstream. This all takes many hours and some people have even slower digestions, often due to a lack of sufficient body enzymes. This is all the more reason it's wise to take a multi-enzyme with each meal. Health stores have a wide variety to choose from. After the food has been broken down into a fine liquid by the digestive tract, it still hasn't been absorbed by the body. The liquefied food then must move past little tissues known as "villi" that line the intestines. The suckers of the tiny villi then draw nourishment into the blood.

You Need Go-Power in the Morning!

Again, we must emphasize that this entire process takes hours – so if anyone says that you get immediate strength from eating a heavy breakfast, you know they are totally ignorant of the facts of digestion! You may say, "Yes, that's very well but I'm hungry in the morning. I get up hungry!" We will have to answer that you are all wrong – your stomach has been conditioned to load up with food in the morning. What you mistake for hunger is simply a reflex action enforced by a long-term habit of eating a big, heavy breakfast! Once you discard breakfast and begin to live on the "no breakfast" plan, you will never again put a heavy amount of food into your stomach in the morning. A heavy breakfast makes you sluggish and sleepy just when you need go-power to start your day!

Morning is the time to drink fresh fruit juices or the Bragg Pep Drink or eat the fresh fruit whole. Remember that organically grown is healthier! This is ideal nourishment for early morning because fruit requires the smallest amount of digestion. The natural sugars of fresh fruit provide you with more and better blood sugar energy than any amount of eggs, meat, toast, donuts or coffee. Your body needs blood sugar to operate properly and a healthy person manufactures about half of a thimble daily. This blood sugar is what powers your muscles. Fruits are light and do not require the tremendous amount of nervous energy to digest that heavy foods require! We have seen people banish many physical problems after going on the "no breakfast" plan, combined with a good diet featuring plenty of fresh organic fruits and vegetables and their juices!

Health Miracles are Within Your Power

Now you have a complete overview of the Toxicless Diet, Body Purification and Healing System: the "no breakfast" plan, a water-only fast 1 day weekly and progressively adding more fresh fruits and raw or lightly cooked vegetables to your diet. When you reach the point where you have fully embraced these principles, the New You will appear! You will feel completely different! You will have more energy, endurance and go-power! You will sleep easier and wake well-rested after sleep. Those nagging aches and pains that have troubled you will fade away. Your eyes will become clearer and your skin more youthful. These are the rewards you will receive when following Mother Nature and living by her wise laws!

When you live The Bragg Healthy Lifestyle you can help activate your own powerful internal defense arsenal and maintain it at top efficiency. However, bad, unhealthy eating habits and lifestyle make it harder for your body to fight off illness! – Paul C. Bragg

Nutrition directly affects growth, development, reproduction, well-being of an individual's physical and mental condition. Health depends upon nutrition more than on any other single factor. – Dr. Wm. H, Sebrell, Jr.

Nature, time and patience are the three greatest physicians. – Irish Proverb

Nature never deceives us; it is always we who deceive ourselves. – Jean Jacques Rousseau

Young men in their 20s who are 20 pounds or more overweight nearly double their chances of developing osteoarthritis of the knee and hip in later life, according to a long-term study of graduates from the Johns Hopkins School of Medicine. – UC Berkeley Wellness Letter

Be Aware of These Health Dangers!

Keep World's Plant Seeds Alive – Not Sterile!

Until recently the magic of the garden, the joy of growing plants and food, was as simple as collecting Mother Nature's seeds and caring for them season after season. Since I was 5 years old I have taken great joy in collecting seeds and giving them away, spreading the beauty of the plants they contained throughout the world. My Dad filled me with wonder at the stories of Johnny Appleseed's accomplishments (see page 30 & 104), and I strive to follow his admirable path. Sweetpeas were my favorite. My Dad and I gave away thousands of sweetpea seeds and they are all over the world. Now simple human pleasures as this are in jeopardy. Some large seed companies now claim their seeds as "intellectual property." In this way, seed companies prohibit farmers by force from saving and reusing seeds from one crop to the next. Even more disturbingly, in recent years major seed companies have made great strides in genetically engineering sterile seeds that sprout plants incapable of reproducing (see page 104 – Terminator seeds). If Dad and I didn't collect and spread these sweetpea seeds around the world, there would be no seed legacy to give us joy. These seeds would be no more than rotting pellets in the ground. Save the world's seeds – for you and your children! Write your elected representatives – protest with strong words that you want this stopped! Make your voice heard! See website: www.rafi.org/usda.html

The Facts About Deadly Vaccinations – Don't Get Them

42

Most in the western world today think of vaccinations against infectious disease as the great miracle of modern medicine. Unfortunately the sad truth is vaccines pose too many health risks. But a growing number of doctors are now warning that there is a correlation between the rise in vaccine use and the growing incidence of asthma, allergies, cancer, chronic fatigue syndrome, attention deficit disorder, autism and many other ailments. Demand your rights to protect your children from compulsory vaccinations (all states permit religious exemption, except Mississippi & West Virginia). Call 505-983-1856 and for $4 get a sample exemption affidavit and a copy of the exact laws of your state. Submit this affidavit to school nurse and check off "religious exemption" box on school form. Learn more about this grave health risk at these informative websites: • home.sprynet.com:80/sprynet/Gyrene • 909shot.com • tetrahedron.org *or read these shocking books:* What Parents Should Know About Immunization *by Jamie Murphy* • Vaccines: Are They Really Safe and Effective? *by Neil Z. Miller* • Vaccination & Immunization: Dangers, Delusions & Alternatives *by L. Chaitow. Order books 505-983-1856*

Beware of Deadly Aspartame Sugar Substitutes!

Although its name sounds tame, this deadly neurotoxin is anything but. Aspartame is an artificial sweetener (over 200 times sweeter than sugar) made by the Monsanto Corporation and marketed as "Nutrasweet," "Equal," and "Spoonful" and countless other trade names. Although aspartame is added to over 9,000 food products, it is not fit for human consumption! This toxic poison changes into formaldehyde in the body and has been linked to migraines, seizures, vision loss and symptoms relating to lupus, Parkinson's Disease, Multiple Sclerosis and other health destroying conditions (even Gulf War Syndrome). Learn more information about this crime against our health. Check website: aspartamekills.com and holisticmed.com/aspartame/

Chapter 4

Your Transition Diet Fully Explained

You are on Your Way to a Miracle!

We want you to thoroughly understand that the Toxicless Diet, Body Purification and Healing System is not made up of special diets for specific ailments. There are no special diets given. It is based on the simple principle that the body will naturally heal and maintain itself after the individual begins to follow The Bragg Healthy Lifestyle which eliminates the deeply buried toxic poisons, obstructions and encumbrances that have been accumulating in the body for years. If any drugs have been taken, residue of these chemicals will still be buried deep in the spongy organs and tissues of the body and must also be removed before they cause trouble.

43

During the time my father suffered from TB as a teenager he was given enormous amounts of powerful drugs. It took him many years to eliminate those drugs from his tissues through fasting and living closely to Mother Nature! He went through a number of healing crises in those years before he was totally free from the vicious drugs given to him. Read our book *The Miracle of Fasting* (see back pages for our book list). It has inspired millions of Russians to live a healthy lifestyle – it's been #1 in Russia for over 14 years now! This life-changing, humble book has altered the lives of millions worldwide – from the Beach Boys, who over 30 years ago used our teachings to get off drugs and alcohol, to Dick Gregory, who went from an unhealthy 350 pounds to a lean, healthy 150 and has run in 8 Boston Marathons!

The Toxicless Diet, Body Purification and Healing System goes directly to the root cause of your physical problem. The System has no interest in the symptomatic effect of an individual's ailments. Sadly, most people just

than deal with the root cause of their ills. Please read our book, *Build Powerful Nerve Force*. We feel that everyone will benefit from this text. We believe that most all physical problems are caused by an excessive accumulation of toxic waste and poisons from unhealthy foods in the pipes and organs of the body. We also believe only a combination of a healthy, natural diet and consistent fasting (1 day weekly) will flush these long-buried poisons out of the body.

We do not believe that physical problems are caused by tension, stresses or emotional upsets. A strong, clean and toxin-free body can beat most all health problems! Some people will say that all their problems are due to nerves. This is rubbish! Healthy nerves that are free of toxic poisons can meet almost any crisis. Again, we stress reading our book on how to *Build Powerful Nerve Force*. Many people with deep-seated physical problems want to blame everything on an outside agent. When you start this program you must first admit that only you are responsible for your physical condition, and that you alone are solely responsible for improving yourself!

Only Mother Nature and You Can Cure You!

Some people may have brought on their troubles because they were ignorant of the great Nutritional Laws of Life dictated by Mother Nature. Others realize that following The Bragg Healthy Lifestyle is the single most important factor in regaining and maintaining their health! But many will lack the inner strength to battle their false desires for unhealthy, refined, processed, sugared, dead foods and will continue to build up the poisons in their bodies with their unhealthy lifestyles!

Each individual must face the fact that only through their own daily constructive, healthful actions can they heal themselves! This is a cold, hard world! Everything in this life has a price! If you want Higher Supreme Health and wish to prolong your life, you must pay the price with dedicated, hard work! This means faithfully following a natural healthy diet and being consistent

44

with your weekly 24 hour cleansing fast. We fast every Monday and the first 3 days of every month. Our fast days provide us with more leisure and free time as our body works at "cleaning house"! Try it, you will love it!

Internal Purity Promotes Youthfulness

The energy and vitality of a young child can be yours at any age when you choose to follow Mother Nature's and God's Eternal Laws of Life. Following this System provides you with the vitality of youth, because youthfulness is Internal Purity! Total Health is not a matter of age, but it's a matter of Internal Perfection!

My father, when heading towards a century, was physically younger than a fit man of 40! We do not live by calendar years. We live in biological years and this is what counts! How clean are your arteries and veins? How are your blood pressures? Ours are 120 over 60 like healthy youngsters. We both have a steady, strong pulse of 60. We have strong eyes and ears that hear every sound. We are not interested in birthdays! We concentrate on living our Bragg Healthy Lifestyle which keeps us internally cleansed, healthy and youthful!

You will reap the same benefits my father and I enjoy when you seriously follow The Toxicless Diet, Body Purification and Healing System! But you must be faithful every day and be the healthy captain of your life! This is not a fad diet – most diets are "yo-yo" diets where your weight just goes up and down! The Bragg Healthy Lifestyle is something that becomes a part of you and your daily lifestyle and it's not a diet per se – but a lifelong lifestyle for super health and longevity!

We want you to live a long, healthy, happy, fit life! Decide daily that you want to feel strong, vigorous and that you will banish your aches, pains and tiredness! It's up to you! We pray nightly for all our friends and Bragg readers to be guided down the righteous path of healthy living through these written words – that never tire and can be with you night or day – just for the reading!

Caution: The Army Diet – What you overeat goes to the front.

The Bragg Healthy Lifestyle Promotes Super Health and Longevity

The Bragg Healthy Lifestyle consists of eating a diet of 60% to 70% fresh, live, organically grown foods; raw garden salads, vegetables, fresh fruits and juices; sprouts, raw seeds and nuts; 100% whole-grain breads, pastas, cereals and nutritious beans and legumes. These are the no cholesterol, no fat, no salt, "live foods" which combine to make up the body fuel that creates healthy, lively people. This is the reason people become revitalized and reborn into a fresh new life filled with joy, health, vitality, youthfulness and longevity! There are millions of healthy Bragg followers around the world proving that this lifestyle works!

Natural Health Laws for Physical Perfection

These Natural Laws God and Mother Nature put in motion are wise, perfect laws created for your own good:

- You must eat natural foods and never overeat.
- You must breathe deeply of God's pure air.
- You must exercise the 640 muscles of your body.
- You must give your body pure, safe, clean water.
- You must give your body gentle sunshine.
- You must not overwork or burden your body; this leads to stress, tensions and nerve depletion.
- You must keep the body clean inside and outside.
- You must live by divine intelligence and wisdom.

The human body is a miracle, give it the best. Within us is the inherent potential to become perfect! It is the intent of our Creator for us to have a physically perfect, healthy, happy and peaceful long life!

My father and I have been able to discard all of the civilized world's heavy, refined and processed foods. We love our Bragg Healthy Lifestyle and all the nutritious, delicious, healthy foods. We work daily on our individual internal purity to keep our bodies clean and healthy!

Please decide now to begin your Bragg Healthy Lifestyle Journey to Higher, Total Health for Total Wellness!

"One step is the beginning of a 10,000 mile journey."

Enjoy a Tireless – Ageless – Painless Body
Living The Bragg Healthy Lifestyle

Most people have a dreadful fear of growing old. They are afraid of becoming a burden to themselves, their family and friends. This is not inevitable!.

But do not despair in your golden years – enjoy them! My dad, Paul C. Bragg, said life's second half is the best and can be the most fruitful years. Linus Pauling and Grandma Moses and the amazing Mother Teresa have all proven that! Three famous men – Conrad Hilton, J.C. Penney and foot Doctor Scholl were all Bragg health followers and lived strong, productive, active lives to almost 100. Millions of others worldwide have lived long, healthy lives following The Bragg Healthy Lifestyle.

We teach you how to forget calendar years and to regain not only a youthful spirit, but much of the vigor of your youth. It's your duty to yourself to start to live The Bragg Healthy Lifestyle today – don't procrastinate!

Square your shoulders and look life straight in the face. Keep premature ageing out of your body by following The Bragg Healthy Lifestyle System. You must eat foods that have a high rate of vibration (an abundance of raw, organic fruits and vegetables) and do a water fast one day a week. Also, do some Bragg Super Power Deep Breathing exercises, get 8 hours of restful sleep at night and keep your body relaxed. Don't let anything rob you of your emotional and nervous energy and precious Vital Force. Do read our *Nerve Force* book.

Your body is being made anew every day! Premature ageing and senility result from toxic debris that accumulates when you live an unhealthy lifestyle. Eat right, exercise for good circulation throughout your body, and there will be little or no buildup of toxins that will clog up and prematurely age your body.

Cultivate and hold onto the spirit of youth and it will be yours! You can feel younger! You can look younger! Keep your spine straight to maintain high energy level. Do The Bragg Posture Exercise (page 110) and follow The Bragg Healthy Lifestyle daily and you'll see miracles!

If you find yourself already in the clutches of premature ageing, begin your fight for the return of your youthfulness. Start your own health crusade today to restore this priceless possession! We have faith in you! You can do it!

Train your body as an athlete would. Follow our clear, concise instructions and soon you will regain strength, virility, energy, vivacity and enthusiasm! Enjoy that most precious of all earthly gifts – the power and joys of youthful, healthful living. Men and women can become more youthful no matter what their age! Go for it! You can retain the spirit of youth beyond the century mark, just like the Hunzas and Georgians of Russia are still doing!

Today Start to Detox and Flush the Toxic Poisons Out of Your Body!

1. Eliminate the toxic foods of civilization from your diet forever! See page 23 for the foods to avoid list.

2. Complete a water-only 24 hour fast every 7 days. Our book *The Miracle of Fasting* has more information you need to know on this tremendous subject. You will extend your life, plus save 15% off your annual food bill! Read pages 84-99 for more fasting information.

3. Eliminate breakfast. If this proves too difficult, have only fruit juice and/or fresh organic fruit, perhaps with some raw wheat germ and honey or try our Bragg Healthy Pep Drink. Some people are so habit-bound to a big breakfast that it takes a little time to eliminate this unimportant meal. If you still feel you need more in your stomach in the morning, try a dish of whole grain cereal or an egg with a few slices of whole grain toast. But always remember that a heavy breakfast is the most useless and energy-robbing meal of the day!

Every morning upon rising have your Bragg Apple Cider Vinegar and Honey Cocktail. Mix 1 to 2 teaspoons of Bragg Organic Raw Apple Cider Vinegar (with the "Mother") with an equal amount of raw honey in a glass of distilled water (diabetics should omit the honey). Please read our book *Apple Cider Vinegar – Miracle Health System* for more insight into this miracle health tonic.

You Will Gain Super Energy

When you give up breakfast you will be thrilled and have all the more Super Energy to enjoy! In our personal lives, my father and I do most of our creative work in the morning. And when it's time for our daily physical activity – such as hiking, swimming, tennis or other sports – we are still filled with vital strength. Remember, it takes a tremendous amount of energy to digest a heavy breakfast. You cannot put your energy in two arenas at once, into both food and activity. People often wonder why we accomplish so much between 6 a.m. and noon. It is because we have not dissipated our Vital Force on a big breakfast. Our daily Apple Cider Vinegar Cocktail, whole or juiced fruit or the Bragg Healthy Pep Drink is all we ever need – and we both have inexhaustible super energy!

You Must Earn Your Food

4. By noon you are ready for the first meal of the day. You have earned it. You have used both mental and physical energy. Always start this first important main meal with a large health salad consisting of coarse vegetables – all raw (grate finely if chewing problems, etc.). Make the base of your health salads from "Nature's Broom" veggies – chopped or grated cabbage, carrots, beets and celery. To this base you can add any fresh, raw vegetables you desire: broccoli, cauliflower, turnips, cucumbers (with their unwaxed green skin), lettuce, radishes, parsley, peas, avocado, tomatoes, green onions, mushrooms, red and green peppers or any other fresh, raw vegetables. See salad recipe page 115.

Top this wonderful mixture with a fresh salad dressing made of Bragg Organic Raw Apple Cider Vinegar (with the "Mother" enzyme), honey and virgin olive oil. You can find the recipe on page 115. Always eat your fill of raw salad first! Never let hot food touch your mouth until you have finished your health salad! The salad is the internal broom, purifier and strong fighter that pushes toxins out. Toxins just have to move out of the body when the nutrients of these raw salads get to work.

You are what you eat, drink, breathe, think and do. – Patricia Bragg

Eat Slowly – Chew Thoroughly

If you have not been used to eating a large raw vegetable salad, go slowly! Eat slowly and always chew thoroughly. Remember that your stomach has no teeth! You may say to us, "Raw salad fills me with gas" or "Raw salads do not agree with me." We can only answer, "The salads agree with you, but you don't agree with them!" When a salad does not agree with you, it shows you have sluggish, unhealthy bowels. In that case there is only one thing to do – gradually change and move at the speed that fits your condition! Slowly you will improve to gracefully accept these nourishing salads. Remember, the salad is the master internal cleanser and "Mother Nature's Broom!"

People with bad dentures or loose teeth, the sick, even toddlers who need nutritious salads, but can't chew well, it's best to finely grate or blend their salad – it's delicious.

Everyone is different and this is why you should keep a daily journal recording your food intake and your reactions for: mucus, headaches, eliminations, energy levels, mood swings, sleep patterns, etc. Start today!

5. What to eat after your salad? The best would be freshly cooked vegetables like lightly steamed greens, cabbage, stringbeans, peas, corn on the cob, carrots, beets, broccoli or any vegetables desired and a baked potato, some whole grain pasta, brown rice or lentils, etc.

6. Now what about protein? If you feel you need meat, eat it. Just remember, on this diet you do not eat meat more than 2 to 3 times a week and that you can always have the delicious vegetable proteins such as brown rice, tofu, beans, lentils, raw nuts and seeds. If you have bad teeth the raw nuts might be better ground or taken in the form of nut butters . . . the same with raw seeds like sunflower, pumpkin and sesame. It may be best to eat them ground. Buy a $20 coffee grinder to grind your raw nuts and seeds.

Many times we make a big raw salad for lunch and we finish off with a few pieces of dried fruits such as sun-dried dates, raisins, figs and some raw nuts.

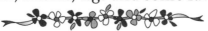

If you truly love Nature, you will find Beauty everywhere. – Vincent Van Gogh

7. Don't worry about getting protein. Traces of protein are found in all foods. Just think, mother's milk is only 3.5% protein and a new human body is built with this small amount of protein. We never worry about getting our daily quota of protein. The body is a miracle chemical factory and can easily convert other foods into protein. We don't believe in heavy animal protein diets! For over 50 years we've heard doctors and nutritionists declare the value of high-protein diets. But in our health work, we've found that many who did high-protein diets got into serious trouble (high blood pressures, heart trouble and strokes, gout, kidney, prostate and liver disorders).

Racehorses are Vegetarian Winners!

The racehorse does not eat concentrated protein. They get their great speed, strength and endurance from the vegetable kingdom. You can also eat raw nuts, seeds, raw wheat germ, brewer's yeast, natural brown rice and beans which are all wonderfully rich, healthy sources of non-cholesterol and non-uric acid protein.

You must always keep in mind that meat is a secondhand food. The animal ate the green growing things that produced the meat. And when that animal was killed, it's flesh retained all the poisons that it had within its body! We have told you that meat has uric acid and contains heavy concentrations of visible and invisible saturated fats! Remember these are the waxy fats (cholesterol) that will clog and plug up the human pipe system and the vital organs!

Unhealthy Gums Cause Tooth Loss

Millions lose their teeth due to unhealthy gums (pyorrhea) due to mushy, refined, sugary diets. A healthy lifestyle promotes healthy gums. Also daily apple cider vinegar gargles (1 teaspoon ACV in ½ glass water) and finger massage the gums (massage upper gums down, lower gums up).

Beware of Toxic Silver (Mercury) Fillings

If you have any silver amalgam fillings in your mouth, have them carefully removed. Replace them with safer, non-toxic composites. For health minded dentists in your area call (407) 298-2450. They will give you the names of dentists in your area. Or see website: iaomt.org/how.htm

Meat Clogs Arteries and Veins

We know many people around the world eat meat. But in America, Australia, New Zealand and the United Kingdom, people consume larger amounts of meats in their daily diet. We also know that one out of every two deaths are caused in these countries by heart disease. Heart specialists agree that the waxy, saturated fats of meat are the main cause of clogged arteries and veins!

We never try to make our health students and readers vegetarians. The choice must be yours! We believe that by properly combining the natural foods, people can, if they strongly desire it, eat meat 2 to 3 times a week and still live a long, healthy life. Try to get only meats that are fed healthy and are hormone-free and drug-free, etc. But we believe that the daily, heavy meat eaters can get into serious health and heart trouble! Be health wise – vegetarian meals are healthier! Fact: vegetarians live healthier and longer! Also forget milk and milk products! Studies show serious health problems started with pasteurization of milk. (See web: notmilk.com) We suggest you use soy or Rice Dream milk (vanilla flavor tastes best) – both are delicious and nutritious!

We have told you that the ideal diet of man is the one he lived on in the warm, tropical Garden of Eden. Now man lives everywhere and he must adapt himself to his particular climate. We do not believe it is possible for a person who is living in a cold climate to eat as if he lived in the tropics. Unless the fruits and vegetables are readily available, and he has conditioned his body and bloodstream to the climate, he must eat plenty of beans, brown rice, raw nuts and seeds to build a bloodstream that will keep him warm and healthy. Remember, your diet must fit with your climate!

Please keep the basic principles of The Bragg Healthy Lifestyle in mind at all times and keep adding more raw fruits and vegetables to your diet. Remember, fruits and vegetables are the great purifiers and the detoxifiers. Also buy organic when possible – it's the best in nutrition! Ask your green grocer to buy and stock organic produce!

Over-Fueling the Body is a Slow Killer!

Some people eat as though they were going to do the hardest kind of physical labor! A sedentary person – by habit and conditioning – will get up in the morning and eat a heavy breakfast of cooked or dry cereal, hot cakes with bacon, eggs, buttered toast and a stimulating beverage like China tea, coffee or mucus-forming milk. Wild animals never drink milk after they are weaned. Only domesticated animals will, but vets advise you not to give milk to your pets. We do not approve of milk drinking by adults – neither raw nor pasteurized. It is amazing how you will have less mucus, runny noses, postnasal drip, etc., once you cut milk and its products from your diet. Your daily journal will provide proof of the changes happening to your human machine!

These same people then go to work in an office, store, etc., and sit or stand around. They will usually have a mid-morning snack and then at noon they will eat a heavy meal: bread, meat, a dessert and a beverage like a sugared soft drink or coffee. In the mid-afternoon they again have snacks and more sugared drinks. Then at home they have their biggest meal of the day; consisting of meat, potatoes, bread, dessert and a beverage. Typically they end their day watching TV – while eating another snack! This kind of daily habitual over-eating is making millions of sick, fat, exhausted people. This habit is sending them to doctors, clinics, hospitals and too many to an early grave! Sad Facts: millions are sick and grossly overweight and it's all due to unhealthy lifestyle habits. (See page 107.)

The average person living the ordinary, inactive life cannot possibly burn up tremendous amounts of food! So what happens to people who eat this way? You know as well as we do that they are sick or half-sick for most of their entire lifetimes. They fill the doctors' offices, pharmacies and hospitals with all their health problems brought on by their unhealthy lifestyles. Millions more end up in mental institutions and in old people's homes.

*Nature cannot be hastened. The bloom of a flower
opens in its own proper time.* – Paul Brunton

Overeating is a vicious and dangerous habit! Most people also over-fuel with the wrong foods! They have been told they must have regular meals at regular hours and they believe this nonsense! They hardly have one meal down before they are beginning another. They think that with this constant stuffing they are "keeping up their strength" – but they are doing just the opposite! They are weakening their precious Vital Force! How? By overeating they are burdening the machinery of their entire body! This continual eating also never gives their machinery time to repair or rest. That's the reason we stress a weekly, 24 hour cleansing fast as essential! This is vital to unclogging and cleansing your system! See Chapter 9 for more details on the importance of fasting, plus do read our Bragg book *The Miracle of Fasting*.

We see these greatly over-stuffed and over-fueled people every day. Look around – you, too, will notice many overweight, sluggish victims of over-fueling on the wrong foods! Most of them also suffer from poor posture and chronic fatigue! They get up tired and go to bed tired! They push all kinds of stimulants (coffee, sugars, cola drinks, alcohol and pills) into themselves to try to keep going during the day. Then they swallow sleeping pills to try and get to sleep at night! What a pitiful plight the average person gets himself or herself into! If this describes you, take notice and change your lifestyle towards health today! Don't waste another precious day – start now on your Bragg Healthy Lifestyle!

The Ignorant Ridicule the Health-Minded

These same half-dead creatures are always ready to say cruel things! They ridicule those who strive to take better care of themselves by becoming the "Health Captains" of their health and taking constructive control of their own lifestyles! Please be strong and ignore them!

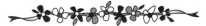

You are encircled by the arms of the mystery of God. – Hildegard of Bingen

During your weekly 24 hour fast try to avoid criticizing anyone or anything! Fill yourself only with loving, positive thoughts, not only on your fasting and cleansing days, but everyday! Before you speak put your words to this test: Is it good? Is it kind? Is it necessary? – Patricia Bragg

People like us are called "fanatics," "food cranks" and "health nuts." The big producers of modern refined and dead foods are largely responsible for these unfair remarks about people who have become vitally interested in good nutrition, natural living and alternative health practices! If living by the wholesome Laws of Mother Nature and God is being a fanatic . . . then we will lay claim to being the biggest fanatics in this whole wide world! We guard our health and will continue to do so throughout our entire, long lives! We love being Health Crusaders and inspiring our readers to attain Total Health and enjoy longevity!

When you decide to follow the Toxicless Diet, Body Purification and Healing System you should not necessarily tell your relatives, in-laws or friends! It is strictly a personal matter until you are on The Bragg Healthy Lifestyle 100% and can then demonstrate its incredible health benefits! Tell only the ones whom it is absolutely necessary to tell when you begin. The average person who stuffs three big meals a day into their stomach thinks illness, premature old-age and death are something that is out of their control.

We call many of these people "the uninformed, unthinking living dead!" They are full of internal body corruption! They are so toxic – so filled with internal clogging – that they are most often negative towards any positive lifestyle changes that will take effort, time and willpower. They will have a flush of youth in their early years and then they will start to decline after 30.

We never argue with these "living dead"! We never allow ourselves to be affected by, or to sink down to, their negative mental attitude. We know what the Toxicless Diet, Body Purification and Healing System has done for us. We know what it has done for the entire Bragg family – the children, grandchildren and great-grandchildren. Why should we waste our precious energies trying to convince some toxin-loaded, willfully health-ignorant person who could care less about the value of good nutrition and living a healthy lifestyle? There are millions of deserving people out there who we are reaching with our health message.

More About the Transition Diet

Now we come to the evening meal. There should always be at least 4 to 5 hours between each meal. The digestive system must have time to do its important work efficiently. The evening meal must start with some kind of fresh vegetable salad or raw fruit. If at the noon meal you had a large raw vegetable salad, now you might want a different raw salad. Maybe you would enjoy just a large cole slaw (grated or chopped cabbage) salad; a cabbage, raisin and carrot salad or a raw grated beet and cabbage salad. There are so many healthy salads a person can select! We have 54 salad and 23 salad dressing recipes in our 448 page *Bragg's Complete Gourmet Recipes* book and hundreds of easy-to-prepare, tempting, delicious, healthy recipes to help you make your meal planning easy and fun!! See back pages for book list.

Many people like to change occasionally from the raw vegetable salad to some kind of fruit salad. This is perfectly fine since a delicious fruit salad is not only tasty, but it is a real toxin fighter! Fresh fruits are very aggressive. They will help dissolve and flush toxic poisons out of the body. You should eat your fruit salad at the first part of the meal. Our principle is always to eat something raw at the beginning of meals. But when you eat a fruit salad at the beginning of the meal you should always wait 10 minutes before you start eating your hot food. Fruit leaves the stomach very quickly and prepares the way for the hot foods.

You may now have 2 cooked vegetables – one of them should be of the yellow variety and the other of the green variety. You could have a dish of lightly steamed or baked carrots with a dish of steamed greens such as chard, kale, spinach, mustard or turnip greens. These yellow and green vegetables are rich in the very essential vitamins, minerals and other wonderful nutrients.

It's important that you control how much of the stimulating foods (meat, fish, eggs, cheese and dairy products) you are going to add to your diet. Remember that your body requires only a small amount of protein. No one in the whole wide world can tell you exactly just how much of these animal foods you can tolerate. Protein foods (meats, fish, eggs and dairy products) should be used with great discretion. If you want to use healthy vegetarian proteins at this meal, you may. Personally, we prefer a healthier vegetarian menu without any meat, fish or fowl. Try this for 3 to 4 days and you will soon note the benefits in your journal!

If you crave a sweet after a meal, you may have fresh baked apples, stewed fruit or an occasional health pie, pastry, cake or cookies made with whole grain flour and honey for dessert. You will enjoy our recipe book – it contains hundreds of healthy dessert recipes. It's best to avoid the daily habit of desserts, however, as it's just another form of overeating! After you have had enough to eat – stop! Forget desserts, only have them once or twice weekly or on special occasions as a treat!

"Good Earth" Founder Thanks Bragg Books

Bill Galt, the founder of The Good Earth Restaurant chain, charged himself with Super Health and changed his entire life after reading our books *The Miracle of Fasting* and *Bragg's Complete Gourmet Recipes*. His entire family began to follow The Bragg Healthy Lifestyle. Soon their friends and associates wanted to know what was the cause of

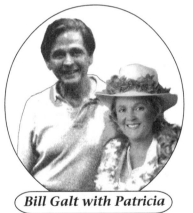

Bill Galt with Patricia

the miraculous changes they saw in the Galts! Their friends wanted what they had – Super Health! Bill and his family started a tiny restaurant that served only lunches. An overnight success, they were soon serving a full menu all day long! Soon they expanded their base of operations and opened a chain of health restaurants, all serving delicious food based on The Bragg Healthy Lifestyle! We are blessed to have a Good Earth Restaurant in Santa Barbara. Many Hollywood Stars often eat there, including the Jack LaLannes. Lucky us! It's nearby, only minutes from the Bragg Health Crusades Headquarters.

Learn to Simplify and Enjoy Your Meals

Eating should be one of the greatest joys of life! There is a rule we follow in the Bragg home: Always get up from the table feeling you could eat just a little more. Remember that you can also overeat on good, healthy food! The simpler the meal, the better! Most animals live on a mono-diet; that is they eat only one item of food at each meal, and they rarely suffer from the digestive distress man suffers from. Modern man often desires to overindulge with the six-course dinner or the buffet dinner spread, eating too many mixtures and very often overeating, which only compounds the abuse!

Go for simplicity in your eating! You will find that the fewer items of food there are at a meal, the less you are tempted to overeat! Make the meal a happy occasion! If it's getting dark, eat by candlelight and play beautiful, soft music on your radio. Always take time to chew your food thoroughly and enjoy your healthy meals! Mealtime is no time for serious discussion or arguments! It's a pleasurable, healthy-refueling time in your life!

Always remember that what you eat and drink today walks and talks tomorrow – it becomes you! You are building yourself with the food you are eating! Give thanks to God and Mother Nature for your foods before you start to eat! It's good for the digestion to be peaceful and say grace! As you eat, millions the world over will go to bed hungry. Malnutrition and starvation are killing millions this very minute, so be thankful for the healthy food you eat! Be thankful you have been led to The Bragg Healthy Lifestyle that will keep you healthier, stronger and more youthful when you follow it faithfully!

The laws of nature are just, but often terrible. There is no weak mercy in them. Cause and consequence are inseparable and inevitable.
– Henry W. Longfellow

As a single footstep will not make a path on the earth, so a single thought will not make a pathway in the mind. To make a deep physical path, we walk again and again. To make a deep mental path, we must think over and over the kind of thoughts we wish to dominate our lives. – Henry D. Thoreau

It's magnificent to live long if one keeps healthy and youthful. – Harry Fosdick

Paul C. Bragg's South Seas Adventure

I had enjoyed living on my Toxicless Diet, Body Purification and Healing System for many years with great results. Through the years I had progressively increased my intake of raw fruits and lightly cooked vegetables. I had not eaten breakfast for years.

I had fasted faithfully for one 24 to 36 hour period weekly for many years and had taken many, many cleansing fasts – some lasting from 7 to 10 days or longer.

Now I was ready to go to the South Sea Islands and discover if it was possible to live on a 100% Toxicless Diet. I was seeking the Garden of Eden! I gave myself a full year for the experiment. I sailed to Tahiti and based myself there. I also visited the smaller islands around Tahiti and I never stopped living on the Toxicless Diet, Body Purification and Healing System.

My diet was exclusively made up of raw and lightly cooked fruits and vegetables. During this entire year I did not eat fish or flesh of any kind, eggs, grains or any dairy products. I ate some raw nuts and seeds, especially when I took long trips – paddling the heavy outrigger canoe to the outer islands or while climbing mountains.

I daily exposed my body to the gentle early morning and late afternoon sun rays. I was often on lonely, deserted South Sea beaches where I could live at times absolutely nude as Adam and Eve did in the Garden of Eden.

With the pure, clean Toxicless Diet and the warm tropical sun, I became like one of the South Sea Natives. In fact, when people did see me they would never believe I belonged to the Caucasian race! My skin and muscle tone were absolutely without a flaw. My strength, endurance, vitality, energy and vigor were supreme. Never before had I attained the physical and internal perfection that I reached on that South Sea Adventure!

One of the most tragic things . . . about human nature is that all of us tend to put off living. We are dreaming of some magical rose garden over the horizon – instead of enjoying the roses that are blooming outside our windows today.
– Dale Carnegie

Bragg Found Secret to Total Health

Many people who have heard about my South Sea Adventure with the Toxicless Diet, Body Purification and Healing System have asked me the question, 'Why, if you attained physical perfection in Tahiti, did you leave that tropical Garden of Eden?' My only answer is that I had found the true secret to Total Health. I could not keep this life-changing health knowledge to myself! I knew I had to share my discovery with my fellow Americans and the world! I felt that now I had definitely proven that man can attain the highest state of physical perfection. I would have been selfish not to share it.

You can't be selfish and hold on to a great discovery! You must share and teach it. It's only by teaching that you, the teacher, come to know your subject better. I knew that I had been privileged to spend an entire year in the Garden of Eden. Knowing that few people could visit the South Seas like I did, I resolved to help others around the world to create their own Garden of Eden where they live!

The banana, papaya, mango, passion fruit, pineapple, coconut and hundreds of other tropical fruits were abundant in the South Sea Islands. It was easy to grow many varieties of vegetables, especially the great vegetable of the South Sea Islands – Taro – a perfect food.

Since I returned from my adventure in the South Seas, I have travelled around the world 11 times. I've lived in all kinds of tropical, cold and temperate climates, but wherever I am I create my own Garden of Eden. In cold countries I add more natural starch to my diet, such as whole grain bread, pastas, natural brown rice, cereals and other products made from whole grains. I also use more raw nuts, seeds and nut butters. I may even add a few eggs or fish, but basically I don't care for flesh foods; I never did. I was reared on a big farm where I saw blood and slaughter at an early age, and it saddened me!

There have been a few times when I ate meat and fish. I did research among the short-lived Eskimos in the Arctic Circle. If I had not eaten fish I would not be here today! I also studied the Laplanders, who live on reindeer meat. Again, without reindeer meat I would have starved.

The Bragg Healthy Lifestyle Gives You Go-Power, Longevity and Happiness!

We enjoy a clean, healthy diet of raw and lightly cooked vegetables and fresh fruits. We have whole grain products when we want them, along with raw nuts and seeds and their butters, and all the delicious beans and legumes. We thrive on this more healthy, natural vegetarian diet. If we felt our bodies needed flesh foods, we would eat them. But we wish to impress upon you to seek organically fed, antibiotic-free, drug-free and hormone-free meats, if and when you want them. The Islanders my father met when roaming the South Seas occasionally ate cooked and raw fish.

After all, there are no two people alike chemically. That is the reason we must, when presenting this Toxicless Diet, Body Purification and Healing System, give you the basics of The Bragg Healthy Lifestyle.

Always choose the most healthy, natural foods that will give your body the best in health! Remember, organically grown fruits and vegetables are always best. **Keep a daily health journal (8.5x11 notebook.) See pages 112 & 133. Chart the health effects various foods have on your performance, energy, weight, moods and well-being!**

By now we have made you aware that the more organically grown fruits and vegetables – both raw and lightly cooked – you are able to assimilate, the cleaner and purer your bloodstream and body will become! But you must decide just how much meat, eggs, fish and dairy products you want. When you sincerely desire a Painless, Tireless and Ageless Body, you will keep those foods out of your body and thus reap more vibrant health.

When you discard all the devitalized, refined and processed foods you are taking the greatest step towards a healthier, longer life. This alone will help put you in a healthier condition! Your body will become cleaner and healthier as you progressively add more raw and lightly-cooked vegetables and fresh fruits to your diet.

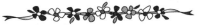

Remember, you are punished by your bad habits of living. – Paul C. Bragg

Have Special Rejuvenating Health Days

We have "Special Health Days" – on these days we consume only fresh fruit and the juice of fresh fruit. Dad and I often do a few days of only watermelon and its juice when these wonderful melons are blood-red, ripe and plentiful. We call this "The Bragg Watermelon Flush" (a great kidney cleanser, etc.). We enjoy going to the beach, lake, river or a mountain resort armed with plenty of watermelons, and feast on absolutely nothing but this fruit for 1 to 3 days. You may also chew and eat the seeds – so nutritious for you! We love to cut the watermelon up and make juice, using a juicer or cheese cloth as a strainer. We put this delicious liquid in a glass bottle and refrigerate. When thirsty after hiking, playing tennis, etc. in the warm sunshine, we enjoy our watermelon juice drink – you will also!

We often enjoy full days of only fresh, ripe fruits, cherries, watermelon, fresh grapes, apricots, etc. Save the apricot kernels (pits), which are high in B-17. Dry, age, then crack and eat 1-2 kernels a day. Very often in our busy lives, we will make it strictly a fruit day. We both seem to work and play harder on our all-fruit day!

62

Of course the heavy meat, egg and refined starch eater might feel sick or feel faint on an exclusively fruit meal, let alone a full day of fruit. The person filled to overflowing with toxic poisons must have their white bread, fried potatoes and meat with plenty of salt. Then they must wash all this down with some unhealthy

---

Living under conditions of modern life, it's important to bear in mind that the refinement, overprocessing and cooking of food products either entirely eliminates or partly destroys the vital elements in the original material.
– United States Department of Agriculture

We are God's work of art. – Ephesians 2:10

True wisdom consists in not departing from nature, but molding our conduct according to her wise laws. – Seneca

---

Bragg's organic raw apple cider vinegar is vital to the body's digestive balance by stimulating the flow of precious enzymes and saliva in the mouth. I recommend for improved digestion you sip ⅓ tsp. before meals to activate the flow of digestive juices.
– Gabriel Cousens, M.D., author, Conscious Eating

beverage like beer, wine, cola drinks, black tea or coffee. Toxin-laden persons shamefully crave the heavy foods they shouldn't be eating. They love heavy gravies, thick meat stews, sugar desserts, pies, jam, jellies and ice cream.

If they stop eating their unhealthy diet of rich, heavy meats, fats, gravies and sugars and replace it with healthy organic fresh salads, vegetables, fruits and their juices, then the much needed toxin-flushing would begin. This cleansing crisis sometimes alarms them. If they are weak in character or lack will-power to follow this healthy lifestyle – they can easily revert back to their unhealthy diet. We pray that all our readers will be strong and follow this Bragg Healthy Lifestyle! We want you to experience this wonderful health and vitality we enjoy!

When the body is clean and purified you no longer crave the rich heavy foods of civilization. When you re-educate the 260 taste buds of your mouth, it is almost impossible to let any unhealthy, toxic foods enter your system. Your clean, newly educated taste buds will refuse to let these foods pass by them. They become the loving, wise guardians of your Holy Temple – Your Body!

63

It never hurts to brush up on the three Rs:
- *Respect for yourself.*
- *Respect towards others.*
- *Responsible living today, tomorrow and always!*

The Y2K Problem Challenges Us All!

On Jan 1, 2000 many computer software programs and imbedded microchips, programmed to identify the year by its last 2 digits, will think it is 1900, causing date-driven computations to fail and computer-reliant systems to malfunction or shut down. In fact, current systems that perform both 2000 forecasting on transactions have already begun to experience failures. If these "year 2000" or "Y2K" problems are not remedied, the disruptions that result could range in delays of airplane flights, to interruptions of phone service, business bankruptcies, power failures, global recessions and civil unrest. It would be wise to store some food and water supplies for a few months in case needed. – Charles R. Halpern, Y2K Advisor

For more frank info on Y2K check out these websites:
- *y2ktimebomb.com* • *survey2k.com* • *garynorth.com*
- *cassandraproject.org* • *y2k.com* • *y2knapa.com*

The greatest antidote to worry, whether you're getting ready for spaceflight or facing a problem of daily life, Y2K, etc., is preparation.
– Senator John Glenn, Astronaut

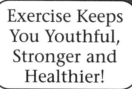

> Exercise Keeps
> You Youthful,
> Stronger and
> Healthier!

Paul C. Bragg and Patricia Lift Weights 3 Times Weekly

Give us Lord, a bit of sun,
A bit of work and a bit of fun.
Give us, in all struggle and sputter,
Our daily whole grain bread and food.
Give us health, our keep to make
And a bit to spare for others' sake.
Give us too, a bit of song
And a tale and a book, to help us along.
Give us Lord, a chance to be
Our goodly best for ourselves and others
Until men learn to live as brothers.

An Old English Prayer

Chapter 5

Questions & Answers About The Bragg Healthy Lifestyle

A Quick Look at Some Frequent Questions

We've traveled the world sharing The Bragg Healthy Lifestyle. We continually tell our health students as well as you, our readers and health friends, that our System is not a set of diets for specific ailments. The Bragg Healthy Lifestyle only recognizes one cause of human suffering and that is the clogging of the pipes and organs of the human body by toxic materials that have been deposited within its tissues due to an unhealthy lifestyle.

We are not in the curing business! We recognize no cures – except those that the body's internal, basic biological functions perform themselves! The body is self-cleansing, self-repairing and self-healing! Your body will do its best work when you do your best to give it a fair chance by following The Bragg Healthy Lifestyle.

Assist Mother Nature in this purification process and your physical problems will soon vanish. This System is not interested in the name of an ailment. We are only interested in what kind of wrong foods and beverages you have ingested and how long you have used them. If you have been saturating your tissues with toxic poisons for years, then you have built up large amounts of toxins which put pressure on your nerves and organs. This can cause aches, pains and worse, premature death!

When students ask us what they should do for a special ailment, we give but one answer, and that is to follow The Bragg Healthy Lifestyle and detoxify! So many people seem to think they should have a special diet for their special physical problem. This is not true. This is not a cure. When the body is cleansed, it releases the toxic poisons and becomes purified . . . then there are no longer distressful toxins to cause health problems!

The Most Asked Questions

Question: *I have suffered from an inflamed colon for years. Raw fruits and vegetables give me terrible gas pains when I eat them. How can I go on this diet since I haven't had raw fruits and vegetables in years?*

Answer: Of course you cannot eat a lot of coarse raw fruit and vegetables at first! You will have to slowly start your program by using soft, mashed, cooked vegetables, stewed fruit such as apple sauce and then gradually add some soft, young, fresh lettuce to the diet. Then a small peeled sliced tomato. Your one day a week fast will help heal and rest your inflamed colon. No food will pass through your digestive tract for 24 hours. This gives your Vital Force a chance to do its healing work. It took you a long time to get into this miserable condition! You must be patient and give your body a chance to heal this raw, inflamed digestive tract. Then have a day where you eat nothing but apple sauce or grated fresh apples. Also use aloe gel (drink 1 Tbsp 3 times a day in juice or distilled water) and the Bragg Apple Cider Vinegar drink on page 114 to soothe the digestive tract and colon.

66

Question: *Can a five-year-old child go on this program?*

Answer: Yes, in a modified way. A five-year-old child is a growing human and therefore must have the growth foods, such as soybeans, brown rice, beans, lentils and tofu. Some fertile eggs, goat's milk and natural cheese are optional. Teach the child to enjoy raw and cooked vegetables, raw vegetable salads and raw fresh fruits along with the nourishing growth foods (see recipes on pg 115). The child of five should have whole grain breads, cereals and pastas. Natural nut butters (but not peanut butter) are perfect foods for the growing child, so is raw wheat germ and honey. A child can easily fast one 24 hour period weekly. The Bragg children fasted one day a week from age three years on. Fast days allowed more time for play, reading and they hardly thought of food on their fast/cleansing days. They always had their Bragg Apple Cider Vinegar drink cold or warm, which they loved.

*Nourish the mind like you would your body.
The mind cannot survive on junk food.*

Question: *My children will not eat raw fruit, raw vegetables or lightly-cooked vegetables. All they want is junk, fast foods – meat, greasy fried potatoes, hot dogs, hamburgers, pizzas, white bread and sweets (candy, cakes, cookies, ice cream, cola, diet and soft drinks, etc). What should I do?*

Answer: It's too bad that these children didn't have a better start nutritionally. Their 260 taste buds have become perverted. They crave stimulating foods: protein, starch, fat and refined sugar products. You will have to take control of their health as a parent and guardian and start to give healthy orders! Keep out of your home the white breads, salty high fat foods, greasy potatoes, fatty foods and the deadly sweets, cola drinks and diet aspartame drinks. (See page 23 for the foods to avoid list.)

Prepare a healthy meal and if they refuse it, that's wonderful – let them fast! Keep them home and confined until they do eat healthy foods. Children need strict discipline in their eating! When they develop a real natural hunger they will discover the goodness of natural healthy foods. Children from 3 years and up can easily enjoy a weekly 24 hour water or juice fast. After they fast, they will relish salads and natural foods you put before them! We prefer you train them to enjoy healthier vegetarian meals. If you insist, occasionally they can have small portions of organically fed meat or fish with their salads and cooked vegetables. But always have them first eat a large raw vegetable salad before any cooked foods.

It's your adult, mature mind overseeing your child's mind. You can slowly change your meals over to healthy menus and control the eating habits of your family! Remember, parents prepare with their two hands for their family – either Health or Sickness – it's up to you!

Every year I live I am more convinced that the waste of life lies in the love we have not given, the powers we have not used. – Mary Cholomondeley

If you are honest with yourself, you will quickly discover that most of the things we truly love to do in our leisure time are not only simple, but also free and surprisingly healthy. So, instead of rushing out to see the latest film or show, why not watch the sunset? Take a walk in nature alone or with a loved one! Read the Bible, a favorite book or listen to your favorite music!

Question: *Can a man who does hard physical labor live on the Toxicless Diet, Body Purification and Healing System and still keep up his strength?*

Answer: Eating heavy food does not produce physical strength. This is an old wives' tale that seems to live on. Many of our students do the hardest physical labor, yet they thrive on The Bragg Healthy Lifestyle. They have no breakfast. For lunch they may take several whole grain sandwiches and some raw nuts, seeds, vegetables and fruits, or a lunch of salads plus some dried fruits and nuts. Some take a container of whole grain pasta or bean salad. We both have tested ourselves with the hardest physical labor and – outside of eating a few more nuts and sunflower seeds – found we can work twelve hours and still feel peppy at the end. It's a clean body that has strength and energy, not a body over-stuffed with heavy foods! We can climb high mountains even on only water or fruits, trail-mix, nuts and dried fruits.

Question: *When I eat raw fruits and vegetables they bloat me up with gas. I belch and pass a lot of wind. Onions, green peppers and cucumbers especially. Why do these do this to me?*

Answer: That shows you are loaded with toxic poisons. When these cleansing aggressive foods get into your digestive tract they start to clean house! Your weekly 24 hour fast (Chapter 9 on page 85), your "no breakfast" plan and your clean, balanced natural diet will ease this condition. Keep at it, for this diet is cleaning house! Also, try a multi-digestive enzyme and "Beano" to relieve gas problems. Remember this: *"Every healthy horse has gas!"*

Question: *I don't seem to digest raw vegetables or fruits properly. Some pass out just as I ate them. Why?*

Answer: You have a crippled digestive tract! A weekly 24 hour fast and a periodic fast of 3 days will help restore the digestive juices to your digestive tract. We also recommend taking a multi-enzyme with main meals. Also sip ⅓ tsp AC Vinegar before meals. Your digestive system has been badly overworked over the years. The coffee, sugar, starch, heavy meats and fats have weakened it. Now it will take time to restore the digestive enzymes and other digestive juices so that you can handle these important health foods. Be patient – it takes time to rebuild the digestive system! Remember to chew each mouthful of food thoroughly! Your stomach has no teeth! This healthy habit improves digestion and health.

Question: *Is it harmful to take a nap after a noon meal or to go to bed soon after your dinner meal?*

Answer: Children and babies, after eating, often take a nap. Most animals eat, then sleep. Your food digests whether you are asleep or awake. If you have your main meal during the day, and are able to rest afterwards, take a nap. We believe in naps when possible. This nap helps give you two days in one. You will awaken refreshed and ready for the rest of your day and evening. But, you must adjust to what is best for you and your time. In Europe, South America, etc. short nap siestas after lunch are popular. Heavy lunches take your energy – avoid them, instead enjoy salads, soups and fruits!

Question: *I have tried to fast for 24 hours, but I get so weak it's difficult to stay on my fast. I get headaches and feel sick in the stomach and some nausea. What should I do?*

Answer: This should definitely convince you what a tremendous amount of toxic poisons you have stored in the pipes, organs and tissues of your body! You had better go to bed during your first few fasts to give your body complete rest and quiet! This rest will aid Mother Nature in removing the toxic poisons from your body. Remember, when you feel nauseated – drink 2 to 3 glasses of water and throw up! You must not fight it – yield! This is usually a sign you have stomach upset from bile, other acids and toxins dumping in your stomach – and your stomach wants them out. This also can happen from food upsets, morning sickness, etc. When you feel nauseated, usually you will feel relieved soon after vomiting it all out.

We know two things about how to prevent death in middle age: smoking and cholesterol. – Richard Peto, Oxford University

A full stomach doesn't like to think. – Old German Proverb

There is no trifling with nature; it is always true, dignified, and just; it is always in the right, and the faults and errors belong to us. Nature defies incompetence, but reveals its secrets to the competent, the truthful, and the pure. – Johann W. Goethe

Question: *When I fast 24 hours – from dinner to dinner or breakfast to breakfast – time goes quickly. But on my 3 day fast may I have herbal teas to warm and console my stomach?*

Answer: Yes! Herbal teas like peppermint, alfalfa, chamomile and anise, etc., are soothing health beverages and always permissible when you feel you need something warm in your stomach. You may add a small amount of raw honey to sweeten it if desired. Remember, China black teas are not permissible. They contain tannic acid, which is used to harden shoe leather, etc. – so from now on substitute herbal teas. You may also enjoy The Bragg Vinegar Drink (page 114) several times a day (cold or hot) as it's a cleanser and purifier. Also, the juice of a lemon in a glass of distilled water, sweetened with honey is permissible when fasting. Many feel this helps when fasting, while others prefer only pure water. You must discover what is best for you!

Question: *My children suffer from frequent colds and heavy mucus. Will this 24 hour fast help them?*

Answer: Yes! The whole Bragg Healthy Lifestyle is a toxicless, mucusless diet. An important factor to consider is that perhaps your children cannot handle cows' milk and its by-products. Millions suffer with mucus problems because milk is a toxic mucus-former for people of all ages. You may substitute soy, almond or rice milk for cows' milk. These are healthier, richer sources of protein and other nutrients than cows' milk. Occasionally enjoy Rice Dream ice cream – it's delicious and dairy free!

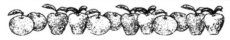

PLAY IT SAFE – USE A VEGETABLE / FRUIT WASH

Before eating raw fruits and vegetables, use this simple recipe to wash and cleanse them of any dirt, bacteria and other toxic matter on the skin: • 1 gal. pure water • ¼ cup hydrogen peroxide • ¼ cup apple cider vinegar. Make several gallons of mixture and store in glass juice bottles for future use. Soak fruits and vegetables in solution for 2-3 minutes in sink or pan. Shake produce in solution to remove any additional contaminants. Now discard solution and rinse produce in pure water. Just because it's organic doesn't mean it's perfectly clean. Remember – many hands touch it before it reaches your kitchen. Play it safe and use this simple produce wash!

Love is the sun shining in us to sparkle our lives! – Patricia Bragg

You Can Reach Mental and Spiritual Heights You Never Dreamed of With a Toxic-Free Bloodstream and Body

Man is a trinity comprised of the Physical, Mental and the Spiritual. It is difficult trying to reach the heights in the mental and spiritual life when the physical body is decaying. The ancient Greeks envisioned man in perfection as having a strong mind in a strong body.

Today millions of people study the Bible daily and benefit from a higher spiritual level. They are truth seekers. They are reaching out for a better way of life but are going about it the wrong way! Before you can become an advanced student in any spiritual and mental philosophy, your body must be clean and free of deadly toxic poisons. Churches should promote fasting.

The great spiritual teachers and philosophers have recognized for over 7,000 years the miraculous cleansing power of fasting. Throughout the Bible, Our Lord Jesus especially showed us the importance of fasting and prayer for those seeking a closer spiritual walk with God! Buddha, Mohammed, Gandhi, the Popes and many other spiritual leaders have recognized fasting as the path to higher spiritual, mental and physical advancements.

71

Paul C. Bragg's Deep Spiritual Awakening

When I went into this work many years ago I had one main goal in mind: I wanted to be well and stay well. I wanted to be healthy regardless of my calendar years! In other words, I wanted a radiantly healthy body with plenty of strength, endurance, vitality and energy to spare for a long, happy life, plus I wanted to share these health truths!

As I attained these goals I realized that the Toxicless Diet, Body Purification and Healing System was opening other channels of thought to me. I found myself searching for spiritual truth. I questioned the religion of my youth. My mental energy was so high that I was able to do a prodigious amount of reading and studying. I sought out brilliant teachers in religion and before I knew it, I was attaining this heavenly serenity and a peace of mind I had never before experienced! My whole personality was changing! I no longer worried and fretted over problems. In fact, I liked the challenges that difficulties presented because I now had, with prayer and the spiritual and mental capacity, a way to look objectively at them and find the proper solution.

Our Creator Teaches You to Be A Good Steward of Your Life, Health, Home, Assets and Family

I found myself a happier person. I found that little things could make me laugh and fill me with joy. I discovered the beauty of the stars at night and of the sky during the day. I enjoyed the rain, the wind and I soon became one with Mother Nature! Since my childhood I had carried many fears and anxieties which I now found were not true problems – they faded as the night fades in the early morning dawn! I was led from the darkness into the light, from the unreal to the real. With my fears and anxieties out of my consciousness I was ready to do bigger things in my profession. I had no fears of traveling any place in the world and delivering my health message. I found I made friends all over the world. I owe this spiritual and mental growth to my healthy lifestyle, prayer time and my walk with God.

I learned to concentrate in prayer and quiet time to anticipate future conditions that I must face. I found answers that saved me countless hours of needless anxiety and worry in the book of life – the Bible!

God gave His creatures light and air and water open to the skies; Man locks him in a stifling lair and wonders why his brother dies. – Oliver Wendell Holmes

Prayer and meditation have been used for thousands of years to quiet the mind and attain inner peace! It can combat stress and confusion. It also helps physical ailments. It has been shown to fight high blood pressure, and can even be done in five-minute versions. Find a quiet place and sit, close your eyes and breathe slowly in through your nose, hold it briefly, then exhale slowly. Focus on health, peace and joy, and a beautiful natural scene. This helps you to center and feel calmer. This technique, with open eyes, can even be done in a traffic jam and can help you go with the flow. – Alan Watts

Where there's great love of God and
Mother Nature there are always miracles. – Willa Cather

Paul C. Bragg Found Peace and Joy

Many people talk about relaxing – just as I used to talk about relaxing – but it was only after years of consistent fasting and purification through diet that I really learned to completely relax! Each day I am able to release all the tensions from my nerves and muscles and thus renew my vitality and energy through complete relaxation. I sleep better now than I did when I was a child! I find that no matter where I am – no matter what the noise or excitement may be – I can sit or lie down, close my eyes and completely relax. This I want for you also!

I find that I am able to understand other people better when they become angry and emotional. I am therefore better able to help them calm down. I feel I am growing – and not only on the physical side! I believe that I am not only building a powerful physical body but, through Cleansing and Fasting, I am also advancing Mentally and Spiritually. I constantly search for light and truth and education along all lines. I find that I have a greater interest in everything that is happening in the world. I find that I understand people better and in understanding others I am able to better understand myself.

This way of life opens many doors that lead to the Higher Life! After all, as we journey through life we should grow Physically, Mentally, Emotionally and Spiritually. Thousands of our students write to tell us of this newly discovered strength in Mental and Spiritual growth they are experiencing. They rejoice when they have found Peace of Mind and the true Joy of Healthy Living!

I am a happy man! I have no worries, no fears and no false ambitions! I lead a simple, happy life and I give thanks for all my blessings daily! I owe it all to the fact that, as my body gets cleaner and purer, I can grow and advance on all three planes of living – Physically, Mentally and Spiritually!

*Nothing transforms anyone as much as
changing from a negative to a positive attitude.*

*Researchers have discovered that the more healthy habits an
individual practices, the longer they live and the healthier they are!
– Elizabeth Vierck, Health Smart*

To desire to be healthy is part of being healthy. – Seneca

Take Time for 12 Things

1 Take time to **Work** –
    it is the price of success.

2 Take time to **Think** –
    it is the source of power.

3 Take time to **Play** –
    it is the secret of youth.

4 Take time to **Read** –
    it is the foundation of knowledge.

5 Take time to **Worship** –
    it is the highway of reverence and
    washes the dust of earth from our eyes.

6 Take time to **Help and Enjoy Friends** –
    it is the source of happiness.

7 Take time to **Love** –
    it is the one sacrament of life.

8 Take time to **Dream** –
    it hitches the soul to the stars.

9 Take time to **Laugh** –
    it is the singing that helps life's loads.

10 Take time for **Beauty** –
    it is everywhere in nature.

11 Take time for **Health** –
    it is the true wealth and treasure of life.

12 Take time to **Plan** –
    it is the secret of being able to have
    time for the first 11 things.

74

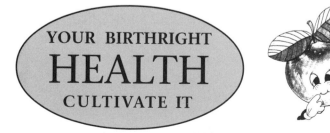

YOUR BIRTHRIGHT

HEALTH

CULTIVATE IT

*Have an
Apple
Healthy Life!*

Teach me Thy way O Lord, and Lead me in Thy plain path. – Psalms 27:11

Chapter 6

Doctor Sunshine – The Gentle Healer

The Importance of Gentle Sunbathing

We believe it is absolutely essential that everyone take every opportunity they can to expose their body to the life-giving rays of gentle sunshine. We also believe that every person must understand the pigment of their skin and not overdo their exposure to the rays of the sun.

We believe that the alpine sunshine – at an altitude of 5,000 feet in the Swiss Alps – played a tremendous part in my father's recovery from tuberculosis. When Dad arrived at Dr. Rollier's Sanatorium, his introduction to sunbathing was supervised closely.

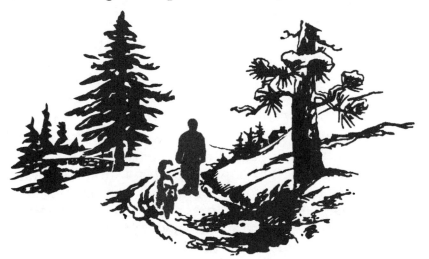

We all grow healthier in nature, gentle sunshine and love!

Nothing in all creation is so like God as stillness. – Meister Eckhart

I learned to listen to my body with an inner concentration like meditation, to get guidance as to when to exercise and when to rest. I learned that healing and cure are active processes in which I myself needed to participate. – Rollo May

Kindness should be a frame of mind in which we are alert to every chance: to do, to give, to share and to cheer. – Patricia Bragg

When Sunbathing Be Wise and Cautious

My father's first day in the alpine sun he only exposed his feet! Each day thereafter the doctor instructed him to expose more of his body to the direct gentle rays of the sun. The conditioning period to expose his body to the sunshine extended over a period of 3 months. By then his body was conditioned to more gentle sunshine.

The doctor believed the best healing rays of the sun were in the early morning and late afternoon. Dad would start his sunbathing program as early as 7 am and enjoy the early rays of the sun. In the cool morning the healing rays were at their highest point. By 11 am they began to disappear and the hot infrared rays took over. This was the time Doctor Rollier advised his patients not to sunbathe. Then after 3 pm they were again allowed to expose their bodies to the gentle rays that had now returned as the hot infrared rays subsided. Try it. You will love the gentle healing rays of the sun.

We believe many people damage their skin by over exposing it too long to the sun's hot, harmful infrared rays. Most people are looking for a tan, so they smear a lot of grease over themselves and expose themselves to the hottest rays, which are the burning infrared rays. There can be no doubt about it – serious damage is done to the skin by this kind of unscientific sunbathing!

Many people have so much toxic acid in their skin that when the rays of sunshine strike those toxic areas, damage is done to their skin. Sunbathing should be done slowly, so that there is no violent reaction on the skin. This means that the safer times to sunbathe are before 11 am and after 3 pm until sundown. You will find that as you detoxify your body and eliminate toxins, you will be able to develop a beautiful natural tan and healthy glow. Most people are so full of toxins that when they go out into the sunshine all they get is severe sunburn. The sun's rays are powerful. We should use them wisely, with great caution and respect! Sunburn can even cause death! Fair people should cautiously do their sunbathing in the early morning and late afternoon gentle rays! Wear sun hats and buy sunscreen SPF 30 from health stores for UVA/UVB protection when needed.

Doctor Sunshine

Doctor Sunshine's speciality is heliotherapy. His great prescription is solar energy. Each tiny blade of grass, every vine, tree, bush, flower, fruit and vegetable draws its life from solar energy. All living things on earth depend on solar energy for their very existence. This earth would be a barren, frigid place if it were not for the magic rays of the sun. The sun gives us light . . . and were it not for light, there would be no you or me!

People who are denied the vital rays of the sun have a half-dead look. They are actually dying for the want of solar energy! Weak, ailing, anemic people are all sun-starved and, in our opinion, many people are sick simply because they are starving for sunshine. For example, older people often suffer from vitamin D deficiency and recent studies show that this nutrient is vital for maintaining, strengthening and repairing human bones.

Sunshine – the Great Healer

The rays of the sun are powerful germicides! As the skin soaks up more of these rays, it stores enormous amounts of this germ-killing energy and vitamin D. The sun provides one of the finest remedies for the nervous person who suffers from anxiety, worry, frustration, stresses and strains. When these tense people lie in the gentle sunshine, its powerful rays provide them with the relaxation that their nerves and bodies need!

Sunshine is a tonic, a stimulant and – above all – the Great Healer! As you bask in the warm, gentle sunshine, millions of nerve endings absorb the solar energy and transfer it to your body's nervous system.

Try this experiment to prove to yourself the value of sunshine in the matter of life and death. Find a beautiful green lawn. Cover up a small space of this lawn with a box, a piece of wood or piece of metal. Day by day you will notice that the patch of grass which was full of healthy rich plant blood (chlorophyll) will start to fade and turn a sickly yellow. Then tragedy happens – the grass withers and dies. Death by sun starvation! Please don't let this happen to you!

Eat Sun-Cooked Foods

The same thing happens to your body when deprived of the life-giving rays of the sun, or when you fail to eat enough sun-cooked foods such as ripe fruits and vegetables. We must have the direct rays of the sun on our bodies and at least 60% of the food that we eat must have been ripened by the sun's rays! When we eat fresh fruits and vegetables we absorb chlorophyll, the rich, nourishing blood of the plant. Chlorophyll is the pure, distilled solar energy that the plant has absorbed from the sun, and is the richest and most nourishing food you can put into your body. **"Chlorophyll is liquid sunshine!"** Green plants alone possess the secret of how to capture this powerful solar energy and pass it on to man and every other living creature. When you get gentle sunshine on the outside of your body and inside your body put 60%-70% daily of organic raw fruits and vegetables, you will glow with radiant health!

We are children of the sunshine! Our life depends upon the sun to produce our food. We can contribute to our bank of health by taking short, gentle sunbaths! If you cannot take a sunbath, then you should at least take an airbath. In the privacy of your own room you can open the windows and allow the fresh air to stimulate the skin of your body – sunbaths and airbaths are special ways that you can add more vitality to your body!

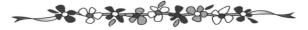

Strongest principle of growth lies in the human choice. – G. Elliot

---

Perhaps the most valuable result of all education is the ability to make yourself do the thing you have to do, when it ought to be done, as it ought to be done, whether you like it or not. – Huxley

---

Don't procrastinate and keep waiting for "the right moment." Today – take action and plan, plot and follow through with your goals, dreams and healthy lifestyle living! You will be a winner in life when you Captain your life to success! – Patricia Bragg

---

Infinite riches are all around you if you will open your mental eyes and behold the treasure house of infinity within you. There is a gold mine within you from which you can extract everything you need to live life gloriously, joyously, and abundantly. – Joseph Murphy

Chapter 7

Doctor Exercise – The Body's Vital Energizer

The Importance of Exercise

You have roughly 640 muscles and all these muscles must be used! If you do not use them, you lose them! If they are not used, they then start to lose their tone, strength and flexibility! Exercise need not be violent and there are hundreds of ways to exercise the human body. The best and greatest of all exercise is walking: no special equipment is required except a good pair of shoes. You can walk vigorously, swinging your arms, for a good workout or just take a stroll. When you walk and breathe in deeply as you stride along you are building Vital Force and stimulating the eliminating and cleansing processes. After walking, swimming is the second-greatest exercise. Any sport that brings into play the muscles of the body can be part of your daily healthy lifestyle. Tennis and even gardening are considered wonderful exercise. You should also have a 20 to 30 minute daily exercise program of stretching, breathing exercises and physical fitness.

The best exercise for the lower abdomen and lower back muscles is to lie on your back and raise both your legs up slowly to a vertical position and hold for a few seconds. Next, slowly lower them until your heels almost touch the floor, then slowly raise back up to a vertical position again. Important: do this exercise slowly and increase the repetitions daily until you can do 30. The best exercise for the internal and external stomach muscles is the sit-up. Lie flat on your back with your knees bent and arms extended over your head. Now return to sitting position and touch your toes. Slowly lower your body back to the floor. Repeat this exercise daily until you are able to do 20 with ease.

It's never too late to begin getting into shape, but it does take daily perseverance. – Thomas K. Cureton

Help for Varicose Veins and Leg Swelling

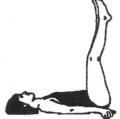

This is good for relieving swollen feet, ankles and legs: lie on the bed or floor and place your feet up on the wall, placing buttocks close to the wall. You can also use the palms of your hands like little irons, gently pressuring legs from the ankles down to the tops of the thighs. This also helps to get any pooled blood and water back into circulation. This brings soothing relief to legs, ankles and also any varicose veins, because it helps recirculate stagnant blood in the legs. After the gentle massage it's ideal to close your eyes for 20 to 30 minutes and listen to music or even take a short revitalizing nap.

Big Muscles Don't Prove You're Healthy!

Just because men or women are athletic or powerfully built with great strength and endurance does not mean that they are internally clean! Far from it. Many athletic people overeat on the heavy, stimulating foods. We know weightlifters who eat 4 or 5 pounds of meat daily, drink quarts of milk and stuff other heavy, stimulating foods into their stomach. They feel it gives them big, powerful muscles and great physical powers. But we have also seen many of those former athletes die in their early 50s and 60s. No, not all athletes necessarily live longer than others! When they stop their heavy exercising – thus slowing down their circulation – the toxic poisons build up from their diet of heavy proteins, fats, refined sugars, etc. This causes an overall slowdown in their protein-burdened body. The toxic poisons are no longer being continually flushed out by the heavy exercising, which they stopped. As the toxins accumulate, they start to suffer from the same ailments that the non-athletic person endures!

Some think it's only strong muscle mass or physical fitness that counts. But it all comes down to the question: "How Clean and Healthy are you internally?"

When you know what you want and you want it badly enough, you will find a way to get it!

Happiness is not being pained in body or troubled in mind. – Thomas Jefferson

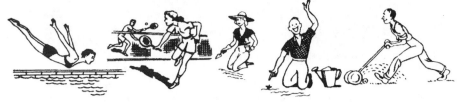

Daily Exercise is a Health Must

We are 100% for physical fitness and exercise! Now, please do not misunderstand us. We think the ideal combination of natural nutrition, multi vitamin-mineral supplements (especially vitamin E) and exercise can work wonders for a person. We love hiking, swimming, tennis, mountain climbing, progressive weight-training and most forms of exercise, plus organic gardening!

Every day of our lives we should look forward to some physical activity. To over-rest is to rust! If you don't use your muscles – your muscles will lose their firmness, tone and strength. But we also realize our bodies must be kept clean of toxic poisons by our weekly 24 hour fast plus, 3 or 4 times a year, a fast lasting from 7 to 10 days.

When you follow The Bragg Healthy Lifestyle, you are filled with inexhaustible vitality and energy! You are like a child who is healthy and you become an active, healthy and happy person. You love life and activity: walking, swimming, biking, gardening, etc. and keep active regardless of your calendar years! You forget your calendar age and become ageless and tireless!

Exercise helps you lose and control weight in two ways. First, by elevating your metabolism you burn more calories. Second, by building muscle – which requires more energy to maintain – you use even more calories. Exercising promotes better elimination and circulation that helps body cleansing!

Self improvements have been shown to be effective to help you accept yourself for what you are and feel positive for what you see in yourself and your future goals! Goals practiced daily for about 15 minutes are more productive than spending all your waking hours fighting to lose weight, or other negatives you find in yourself. During self hypnosis (self-guidance) tell yourself to let go all the bad feelings about yourself, breathe deeply, then relax. Concentrate on feeling comfortable at each area of your body and tell yourself to treat yourself more lovingly. When you can forgive yourself, you'll be able to forgive others easier and feel better about yourself and everyone around you! This will help you become more motivated to improve your lifestyle!

Let me look upward
into the branches
Of the towering oak
And know that it grew
slowly and well.

Give me, amidst
the confusion
of my day
The calmness of the
everlasting hills.

Let me pause
to look at a flower
to smell a rose —
God's autograph,
to chat with a friend,
to read a few lines
from a good book.

Break the tensions
of my nerves
With the soothing music
of singing streams
and gentle rains
That live in
my memory.

Chapter 8

Doctor Super Power Breathing

The Importance of Deep Breathing Oxygen The Invisible Staff and Food of Life!

We are breathing machines and must have oxygen constantly or we will perish! The more oxygen we can get into the system, the cleaner our bodies are going to be and the better we are able to absorb more life-giving oxygen into the tissues! We want you to know we are air-gas machines. We live at the bottom of a sea of oxygen – the atmosphere extends 70 miles above us and exerts a pressure of 14 pounds per square inch. The Latin word "spira" means oxygen, air and then spirit. The breath of God and life that goes to every cell in your body is in fact oxygen and therefore air! Most people are shallow breathers. They get oxygen in the upper regions of the lungs but seldom get sufficient oxygen into the deep lower regions of the lungs. They become oxygen-starved and pale and lack go-power!

Directions for Filling the Entire Lungs With Life-Giving Oxygen

Lie flat on your back, either in bed or on the floor, relax and then slowly inhale through your nose and do not consciously try to move the upper chest or the abdominal region. While you are inhaling, place your hands on your lower ribs, which are known as the floating ribs. Now – if you are breathing correctly – you can feel your lower ribs expand. Slowly take in a long, deep breath. When you feel that your lungs are filled to full capacity with air – then you can slowly expel the breath with a long, lip-pursed sigh.

Breathing deeply, fully and completely energizes the body, calms the nerves, fills you with peace and helps keep you youthful. – Paul C. Bragg

Deep Breathing & Fasting Removes Toxins

Deep Super Power Breathing is our best insurance against germs, bacteria and disease. This deep breathing constantly cleanses and purifies the body. When we exhale, we breathe out toxins and carbon dioxide, which must be eliminated since they are the deadliest poisons the body creates. After expelling with a long, lip-pursed sigh, pause 10 seconds, then repeat routine. A long slow inhaled breath – filling the lower lungs and expanding the lower floating ribs – then expel the air and again pause for 10 seconds; then repeat the entire cycle. Do 15 breathing exercises in the morning and at night.

Deep breathing is the most important function in raising the body to its highest potential! By deep breathing you help remove toxic poisons. Full, deep breaths in and out help to remove and eliminate any encumbrances. The body has a great capacity and need for oxygen! The more air you get in the body, the more toxic poison you burn up and the more vitality you create!

Deep Breathing Promotes New Brain Cells

One of the main solutions to creating more energy and better body and brain functioning lies in healthy foods and healthy lifestyle living. Unobstructed oxygen circulation and maintaining a vital, healthy elasticity of the cells and tissues is vitally important. The Salk Institute for Biological Studies, La Jolla, CA shows that adults do generate new brain cells. Remember, oxygen is also a detoxifier. It's like fasting – it helps to remove toxic poisons throughout the body. The cleaner your body becomes through deep breathing, fasting and an abundance of organic raw fruits and vegetables, the more your energy will increase! With a clean, purified body and an ample supply of oxygen you can enjoy a more youthful, energetic healthful body for a longer life.

Our Bragg book *Super Power Breathing* will show you breathing exercises to help you drive more oxygen into your body for super health, energy and longevity.

The average person breathes in one-half liter of air with a typical, normal shallow breath. But the deep breather (athletes, singers, etc.) takes in much more. In fact, the greatest amount of air that can be breathed in and out of healthy lungs is almost 5 liters (the full capacity of your lungs).

Chapter 9

Doctor Fasting – The Miracle Cleanser, Rebuilder and Life-Saver!

Your Tongue Never Lies

The tongue should be called "the Magic Mirror." The tongue reveals the great amount of toxic poison stored in the body. One of the means a doctor uses to diagnose a person is to say, "Let me see your tongue." When the doctor sees a white-coated tongue, he knows that person is in a highly toxic condition. This is one of the oldest methods of diagnosis used by doctors and alternative health professionals.

Remember that the tongue is one end of a tube that averages 30 feet in length, extending from your mouth to the anus. When the tongue is coated it shows that Mother Nature is trying to stimulate some of the deep buried toxins of the body and help remove them!

Sick people often have heavily coated tongues, plus a bad breath. Now when you fast a few days or go on a strict fruit diet such as apples or oranges you will notice that your tongue becomes coated. The fasting and the strict diet starts to loosen the filthy toxic poisons of the body. The tongue is "the Magic Mirror" not only of the stomach, but the entire mucus membrane system.

You should cleanse your tongue by gently scraping its surface with the tip of a spoon. Begin at the back of your tongue. Gently press down and pull the spoon forward towards your tongue's tip; repeat as necessary until the entire top of your tongue has been cleaned of its toxic coating. You can shake the toxins off the spoon into a saucer to see one of your immediate *fast* results.

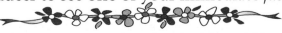

Fasting is the greatest remedy – the physician within. – Paracelsus, 15th century physician who established the role of chemistry in medicine

Daily Tongue Brushing is a Good Habit

After scraping your tongue, use your toothbrush to lightly brush your tongue from the back to the tip (it's a good habit to brush your tongue daily). Then you should gargle with a mixture of 1 teaspoon of Bragg Organic Raw Apple Cider Vinegar in ½ glass of water to rinse any remaining germs or toxins from your mouth. Repeat this cleansing 2 to 3 times a day during a water fast or juice fast. Your body will continue to push toxic slime out the tongue! This tongue coating shows you are doing deep cleansing. It's an accurate indication of the amount of decaying filth, rotting mucus and other toxic poisons accumulated in the tissues of your entire body that are now being eliminated from the inside surfaces of the stomach, intestines and vital body organs.

You can now see by the coated tongue how much toxic poison you have stored in your body. The tongue's surface reveals the great amount of encumbrances that have been clogging up your body maybe since childhood because of unhealthy living and the eating of refined, sugared, high-fat, high-salt, toxic-forming foods.

That is the reason we are not interested in the name of your physical trouble. All physical problems are due to a local clogging of the circulation, tissues and the entire pipe system. If you have a pain in your shoulder and it is inflamed, it could be given the name "bursitis." But we see it only as concentrated toxic poisons at that point. The pain and inflammation are caused from too heavy a concentration of toxic poisons in the shoulder. Naturally there will be inflammation caused by this toxic friction and heavy congestion.

When a person with this condition fasts, the tongue will take on a slimy coating. This shows their body has started to eliminate and push out the toxic waste as soon as they stopped eating. Also, a few days of strict water fasting (drinking at least 8 glasses of distilled water daily) will provide some relief from the pain in your shoulder – depending on the intensity of the condition.

_____

Prevention is always preferable to the cure.

_____

Eat to live, and not live to eat. Many dishes, many diseases. – Ben Franklin

The Human Pipe System
Must Be Kept Clean and Healthy

Let us repeat that every physical problem a person suffers from is the result of constitutional clogging. The entire human pipe system, especially the microscopically small capillaries (the smallest pipes in the body, about the size of a human hair), become "chronically" clogged by the heavily processed, foodless foods of civilization.

There are no special diets that can clean a dirty, heavily coated tongue. This is the reason we give no special diets for special ailments. This is the reason that we do not believe in "cures" of any kind. Only your body is self-cleansing and self-healing when you give it a chance! Daily we pray for our readers to be healthy!

To be well, to stay well and to be free from aches or pains, you must live each day so that you eliminate the toxic poisons you have accumulated over the years. You must also eat right so that you will not build any more toxic poisons and mucus within your body.

The Toxicless Diet, Body Purification and Healing System calls for large amounts of organic raw and lightly cooked vegetables and fresh fruits; weekly 24 hour fasts and periodic fasts lasting from 3 to 10 days. We know what miracles this System of Internal Purification can do for the sick and prematurely old person. So does Professor A. E. Crews of Edinburgh University – who has performed extensive dietary restriction experiments on both mammals and worms – noted on page 93.

We faithfully fast 24 hours every Monday and the first 3 days of each month. We never worry about being overweight – our weight remains balanced and normal! Wait until you experience this miraculous cleansing process! You will greatly benefit from the inner cleansing and will love the pure, clean feeling you receive! For over 80 years my father fasted religiously, as I have since 3 years old, also as millions of our readers and students the world over are living The Bragg Healthy Lifestyle.

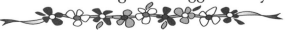

Doubt destroys. Faith builds! – Robert Collier

Purge Your Body of Filthy Toxic Poisons

The characteristics of tissue construction, especially of the important internal organs such as the liver, kidneys, lungs and glands, are all very much like those of a sponge. Now imagine a sponge soaked with a sticky glue or paste. As a person lives on the foodless foods of civilization, the vital organs begin to fill up with this slimy paste or glue (toxic poisons). No wonder they die of horrible diseases of the liver, kidneys and lungs! The vital organs actually become so clogged with these slimy, sticky, decaying toxins that they can no longer function!

Death by toxic poisoning! Death by clogging of the pipe system! Now do you understand why we want you to detoxify, cleanse and purify your body? This is the only natural way to internally cleanse and heal yourself!

We receive thousands of letters yearly from grateful students who have put our Bragg Healthy Lifestyle with fasting to the test and discovered it worked for them! Quite often, when every other method failed them, this lifestyle proved successful! We want to inspire you, our reader and health friend, to improve your whole body, not just to relieve a symptom! We are not interested in symptoms or the name of a bad place in the body! We are interested in your obtaining Super Health and Longevity! We love to hear your successes. Write us!

Fasting – Safe, Effective Way to Detoxify the Body

. . . A technique wise men have used for centuries to heal the sick. Fast regularly and help the body heal itself and stay well. Give all of your organs a rest. Fasting can help reverse the ageing process, and if we use it correctly, we will live longer, happier lives. Just three days a month will do it. Each time you complete a fast, you will feel better. Your body will have a chance to heal and rebuild its immune system by regular fasting. You can fight off illness and the degenerative diseases so common in this chemically polluted environment we live in. When you feel a cold, illness or depression or allergy attack coming on, fast! – James Balch, MD & Phyllis Balch, CNC, Prescription for Nutritional Healing

---

Hollywood Actress Cloris Leachman, a healthy vegetarian who sparkles with health, says, "Fasting is simply wonderful. It's my solution to any problems. I can do practically anything. It's a miracle cure! It cured my asthma!"

Fasting – Mother Nature's Master Healer

Mother Nature heals through FASTING every physical problem that's possible to heal! This alone proves that Mother Nature recognizes but one problem, that in every body the largest illness-causing factors are toxic poisons – decaying mucus, foreign matter, pus and uric acid.

Just look at what happens to people when they suffer from a common cold. They run a high fever (body burning up toxins) while they eliminate great masses of mucus from the sinus cavities of the head, throat, lungs and bronchial tubes. A cold is the body's way of saying, "I must rid the body of this toxic slime to survive!" And a healing crisis is started by the body's Vital Force. Please read all of this chapter twice to let it settle in your mind and inspire you to fast to keep your body healthier!

Colds Push Out Mucus & Toxins – Give Thanks!

The average person who experiences a cold takes absolutely no blame for this condition! Oh no! They will say, "I got my feet wet and caught a cold," "I sat in a draft and caught a cold" or "I caught the cold from a bug my brother brought home from school" . . . Excuses, excuses! They never place the blame on themselves! Three times a day at meals these people load toxic mucus-forming foods into their bodies. They eat ice cream, cakes, candy, soft drinks (with toxic aspartame or sugar), tea and coffee filled with refined white sugar, milk and its by-products which are heavy mucus-formers. And when this mess decays in their bodies they cry out, "I caught this cold, poor me!" Yes, poor ignorant you. You do not catch colds. You eat colds! You develop colds from your unhealthy lifestyle and unhealthy refined diet! See page 23.

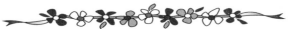

Your body wants mucus and toxic slime out. Do all you can to help remove these toxins. When you feel them in your throat and sinuses cough, spit and blow the mucus out. Your body works hard to collect these unwanted toxins. Please never swallow (recycle) mucus – get it out! Mucus and toxins are trouble-makers and a heavy burden when they stockpile. They can cause future disease and cancers. This is the main reason to live The Bragg Healthy (Toxicless, Mucusless) Lifestyle which promotes a mucusless, toxicless body.

Urine Reveals the Amount Of Toxic Poisons in the Body

The urine shows the amount of toxic poisons in the body. All you have to do is start a strict water fast (nothing else but water). During the days you fast be sure to drink at least 8 glasses of water that has been distilled or purified by reverse osmosis (both of which are pure, delicious, chemical and odor-free). Upon awakening, use a bottle to secure the morning's first urine specimen. Seal the top of this bottle so no air can get in it. Write the date you took the specimen of urine on a label or piece of masking tape and place it on the jar. If you are going to take a 7 day fast, take a specimen upon awakening each morning. Store the dated specimen on a shelf to let it cool and settle!

As it cools and settles you get a revelation before your very eyes. After a week you see the clouds of slimy, putrid mucus. As the days, weeks and months pass, you see before your very eyes the horrible, decaying filth that you eliminated during your fast. These toxins have burdened your vital organs and all your machinery.

90

We have fasted thousands of times in our long careers and we have also kept many bottles of urine from our student fasters. If you looked at them you would hardly believe your eyes. But there is the proof that shows what filth humans carry around with them.

Sometimes we meet some boastful fool who will say, "I eat anything I wish and I am strong and healthy." We simply reply, "You are a walking manure pile! Just fast for a week to 10 days and we will have you flat on your back, stewing in your own decay and toxic poisons that you have piled in your body through the years. These toxins burden your body and – once you start cleaning your system – you will bear witness to the miracles of fasting and its body-cleansing power!"

We have told you that physical strength, athletic ability and physical fitness have nothing to do with basic health. "The stronger they are, the harder they fall" when the body clogs up with decaying toxic poisons.

Infections, Germs, Bugs, Viruses And Bacteria are Human Scavengers

You often hear people say, "A new virus is attacking people. It seems that everyone is picking it up." That is exactly right, since there are thousands of germs floating around everywhere. Remember they are here for a purpose. They are scavengers. They clean up decaying filth. If that decaying filth happens to be in your body, they are going to start eating that toxic slime.

Just remember it is impossible for any kind of germ or virus to attack clean, healthy tissue and an active, healthy immune system! They only eat decaying toxic matter. Personally, we have no fear of infection from any germ or bug. We fast regularly and keep our bodies clean! We eat plenty of organic raw and lightly cooked fruits, vegetables and whole grains. We are very zealous about our health and bodies and therefore we do not put any of the dead foods of civilization into our bodies.

Dirty blood attracts infections! Clean blood is your protection against infection! If you create decaying matter in your body by eating wrong, it is only a part of Mother Nature's plan that germs will come and eat this dead substance! Germs never attack clean, toxic-free tissue or healthy blood!

As a child my father was fed the typical American unhealthy diet of refined white flour products as well as white sugar products such as ice cream, cakes, pies, cookies, jams, jellies, fudges and many foods that were unwholesome and devitalized. He contracted most of the children's diseases – chicken pox, mumps, whooping

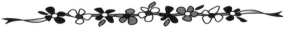

Mind-body techniques can help people take control of their lives and their bodies, but they need to be part of a whole program, including proper nutrition and exercise, to enhance health and well-being. Identifying stress in your life and addressing that issue is essential to good health, and using powerful mind-body techniques like prayer, self-hypnosis and biofeedback are also good for taking charge. These techniques can help the immune system stay strong and heal illnesses.
– Medical Tribune News Service

A strong body makes a strong mind. – Thomas Jefferson

cough and many others. Why? Because his refined, sugary diet put toxins in his body! So the germs came and had a feast on his internal poisons. Now all of the Bragg children are reared on The Bragg Healthy Lifestyle – the Toxicless Diet, Body Purification and Healing System. They never suffer the children's diseases!

Infectious diseases kill many humans. The germs attack the body to eat the decaying toxic matter and many times cause death by destroying vital organs. By following this Body Purification Program you can build a powerful, healthy immune system to keep germs away! Germs eat only decaying matter. Keep clean inside. A powerful and nutritionally fit bloodstream is your greatest defense against the invasion of germs. Germs thrive in a dirty bloodstream and perish in a clean one!

How to Conduct 3 Day, 7 Day & 10 Day Fasts

A fast of 3 days or longer should be conducted under ideal, peaceful conditions. You should be able to rest any time you feel the toxins passing out of your body. During this time you might feel some discomfort. You should rest and relax quietly until the poisons have passed out of your body. It's best to be quiet, at peace and alone when possible. This brief period of discomfort will end as soon as the loosened toxins have passed out of your body through the kidneys, lungs, skin, etc.

During longer fasts do not tell others what you are doing. Why? You must keep only positive thoughts of cleansing and renewing miracles happening in your body. Too often others ignorant about fasting will criticize your fasting with negative comments.

Our fasting is such a very personal and quiet time that many years ago Dad went into the Santa Monica Mountains in California and bought a tract of land in the wilderness of the Topanga Canyon near Malibu where he built a retreat cabin, identical to Thoreau's at Walden Pond near Boston. In that natural seclusion Dad and I enjoyed the quiet peace for our fasting time. If possible, get away to some secluded place to fast in solitude and Mother Nature's fresh air, to enjoy better results!

There are now very fine health spas worldwide where all the conditions are perfect for a restful fast. Inquire at health stores for any in your area. Many of our Bragg students who fast regularly tell us that they use their vacation as a period of fasting and purification of body, mind and soul. Some will rent a place in a quiet country setting to fast in seclusion. It's not necessary to go away from home to fast. Your home is your castle and hopefully you will be more at peace there. The Bragg family are all healthy fasters and, when one of us is fasting, we show consideration for each other. We have an agreement not to ask each other how we feel during the fast. Fasting is so personal that no one can do anything for you during the fast, so the best thing is not to discuss it with others.

When you are on a fast from 3 to 10 days or more, you are really on Mother Nature's miraculous cleansing operating table. Your body is purging the waste, mucus, toxins and other foreign substances out of your body that you had stored from unhealthy, wrong eating, etc.

Fasting Brings Remarkable Results

Professor A.E. Crews of Edinburgh University, who studied both worms and animals, stated: *"Given appropriate and essential conditions of the environment, including proper care of the body . . Eternal Youth, in fact, can be a reality in living forms! It's been found to be possible by repeated processes of fasting, to keep a worm alive 20 times longer than it would have lived regularly. This has also been proven with animals."* Life-extending results have been proven again in a recently published earthworms study. Something to think about, indeed, that proves the merits of fasting! Don't delay – start soon!

Remember, it took time for the body to build up toxins, so it takes time to cleanse and unload them! Take your time! Be faithful to The Bragg Healthy Lifestyle Program. You will reap wonderful, priceless benefits.

Fasting is Cleansing, Purifying and Restful. – Meir Schneider

Everyone has a doctor in him or her; we just have to help it in its work.
– Hippocrates

More Scientific Proof That Fasting Works

Dr. Roy Walford, a famous University of California at Los Angeles Scientist and Life-Extension Researcher is a leading authority in dietary-restriction studies, with over 325 articles in scientific journals. He practices dietary restrictions himself and never overeats. He was the chief scientist of the Biosphere Study in Arizona. This experiment involved 4 men and 4 women living in a totally enclosed environment for 1 year. Their calories were restricted by 29%. During that time they all registered healthier, decreased levels in blood pressure, triglycerides, cholesterol and other toxins! These results were similar to studies conducted by Professor Crews of Edinburgh University on earthworms and animals. For info on Dr. Walford's work on longevity and restriction eating visit his website: .walford.com. To learn more about Biosphere Studies visit: biospherics.org

94

Fasting is based on unchanging biological laws that insist the cause of disease must be removed. After hearing about a natural food diet and therapeutic fasting, individuals may enthusiastically give it a try and get well. It is also possible that they may become excited about the sensibleness of this approach and the prospect of finally recovering their health, but then go home to their friends and family and become discouraged, after being told they would be crazy to attempt such an 'outrageous' treatment. They might even call a few doctors they know, only to be told that fasting is risky, dangerous and stupid.
– Joel Furman, M.D., Fasting and Eating for Health

Those who do good on their own accord shall be rewarded, but to fast is better for you, if you knew it. – Mohammed, 500-600 A.D.

Exercise gurus walk and run daily to maintain their health. A study on leading exercise experts revealed that most did daily walking, some did walking and running, and some played tennis, walked and ran. All stressed 30 minutes a day, six days a week or two to three times a week for an hour each time.
– Sports Medicine Digest

Privation of food (fasting) at first brings a sensation of hunger, occasionally some nervous stimulation, but it also determines certain hidden phenomena which are more important. The sugar of the liver and the fat of the subcutaneous deposits are mobilized, and also the proteins of the muscles and the glands in order to maintain blood, heart and brain in a normal condition. Fasting cleanses and purifies and profoundly modifies our tissues.– Dr. Alexis Carrel

BENEFITS FROM THE JOYS OF FASTING

Fasting is easier than any diet. • Fasting is the quickest way to lose weight.
Fasting is adaptable to a busy life. • Fasting gives the body a physiological rest.
Fasting is used successfully in the treatment of many physical illnesses.
Fasting can yield weight losses of up to 10 pounds or more in the first week.
Fasting lowers & normalizes cholesterol and blood pressure levels.
Fasting is a calming experience, often relieving tension and insomnia.
Fasting improves dietary habits. • Fasting increases eating pleasure.
Fasting frequently induces feelings of euphoria, a natural *high.*
Fasting is a rejuvenator, slowing the ageing process.
Fasting is an energizer, not a debilitator. • Fasting aids the elimination process.
Fasting often results in a more vigorous sex life.
Fasting can eliminate or modify smoking, drug and drinking addictions.
Fasting is a regulator, educating the body to consume food only as needed.
Fasting saves time spent marketing, preparing and eating.
Fasting rids the body of toxins, giving it an "internal shower" & cleansing.
Fasting does not deprive the body of essential nutrients.
Fasting can be used to uncover the sources of food allergies.
Fasting is used effectively in schizophrenia treatment & other mental illnesses.
Fasting under proper supervision can be tolerated easily up to four weeks.
Fasting does not accumulate appetite; hunger "pangs" disappear in 1-2 days.
Fasting is routine for the animal kingdom.
Fasting has been a common practice since the beginning of man's existence.
Fasting is a rite in all religions; the Bible alone has 74 references to it.
Fasting under proper conditions is absolutely safe.
Fasting is not starving, it's nature's cure that God has given us. – Patricia Bragg
         – Allan Cott, M.D., *Fasting As A Way Of Life*

95

Spiritual Biblical Reasons Why We Should Fast
For Healthier, Happier, Longer Walks with Our Creator

3 John 2	Deut. 11:7-15,21	Luke 9:11	Matthew 9: 9-15
Gen. 6:3	Gal. 5:13-26	Mark 2:16-20	Neh. 9:1, 20-24
I Cor. 7:5	Isaiah 58	Matthew 4:1-4	Psalms 35:13
II Cor. 6	James 5:10-20	Matthew 6:6-18	Romans 16:16-20
Deut. 8:3	John 15	Matthew 7	Zachariah 8:1

Dear HEALTH FRIEND,

This gentle reminder explains the great benefits from *The Miracle of Fasting* that you will enjoy when starting on your weekly 24 hour Bragg Fasting Program for Super Health! It's a precious time of body-mind-soul cleansing and renewal.

On fast days I drink 8 to 10 glasses of distilled water, some with ACV (page 114). You may also have some herbal teas and if just starting try diluted fresh juices (add ⅓ distilled water). Every day, even some fast days, add 1 tbsp. of mixture (half oat bran and half psyllium husk powder) to liquids once daily. It's an extra cleanser and helps normalize weight, cholesterol and blood pressure and helps promote healthy elimination. Fasting is the oldest, most effective healing method known to man. Fasting offers great, miraculous blessings from Mother Nature and our Creator. It begins the self-cleansing of the inner-body workings so we can promote our own self-healing.

My father and I wrote the book *The Miracle of Fasting* to share with you the health miracles it can perform in your daily life. It's all so worthwhile to do and it's an important part of The Bragg Healthy Lifestyle.

With Love, *Patricia*

Paul Bragg's work on fasting and water is one of the great contributions to Healing Wisdom and the Natural Health Movement in the world today.
– Gabriel Cousens, M.D., Author, *Conscious Eating & Spiritual Nutrition*

Fasting Cleanses, Renews and Rejuvenates

Our bodies have a natural self-cleansing and healing system for maintaining a healthy body and our "river of life" – our bloodstream. It's essential that we keep our entire bodily machinery from head to toes in perfect health and in good working order to maintain life!

Fasting is the best detoxifying method. It's also the most effective and safest way to increase elimination of waste buildups while enhancing the body's miraculous self-healing and self-repairing process that keeps you healthy.

If you prepare for a fast by eating a cleansing diet for 1 to 2 days, this can greatly facilitate the healing process. Fresh variety salads, fresh vegetables and fruits and their juices, as well as green powder drinks (you can choose from alfalfa, barley, chlorophyll, chlorella, spirulina and wheatgrass, etc.) stimulate waste elimination. Live, fresh foods and juices can literally pick up dead matter from your body and carry it away. Following this pre-cleansing diet, you can now start your liquid fast.

Daily, even during most fasts, we take 3,000 mg. of mixed vitamin C powder (acerola, bioflavonoids, rosehips and C concentrate) in liquids. This is a potent antioxidant and helps flush out deadly free radicals. It also promotes collagen production for new healthy tissues. Also vitamin C and grape seed extract are important if you are detoxifying from prescription drugs or alcohol overload.

A moderate, well planned distilled water fast – our favorite – or diluted fresh juice (35% distilled water) fast can cleanse your body of excess mucus, old fecal matter, trapped cellular, non-food wastes and help remove inorganic mineral deposits and sludge from your pipes and joints. Fasting works by self-digestion. During a fast your body will perform cleansing miracles by intuitively decomposing and burning only the substances and tissues that are damaged, diseased or unneeded, such as abscesses, tumors, excess fat and water and congestive wastes.

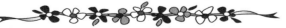

The nation badly needs to go on a diet. It should do something drastic about excessive, unattractive, life-threatening fat. It should get rid of it in the quickest possible way and this is by fasting. – Allan Cott, M.D.

Fasting Accelerates Elimination of Toxins

Even a relatively short fast (1 to 3 days) will accelerate elimination from your liver, kidneys, lungs, bloodstream and skin. Sometimes you will experience dramatic changes (cleansing and healing crises) as accumulated wastes are expelled. With your first fasts you may temporarily have headaches, fatigue, body odor, bad breath, coated tongue, mouth sores and even diarrhea as your body is cleaning house. Please be patient and loving with your miracle human home – your body!

After a fast your body will begin to self-cleanse and healthfully rebalance! When you follow The Bragg Healthy Lifestyle, your weekly 24 hour fast removes toxins on a regular basis so they don't accumulate! Your energy levels will begin to rise – physically, psychologically and mentally. Your creativity will begin to expand. You will feel like a "different person" – which you are – you are being cleansed, purified and reborn. It's an exciting and wonderful miracle that is happening!

Actions speak louder than words and can change your mood if you feel depressed. Take a walk outside – it often helps you sort out and solve your problems. Spend time with a young child – it simplifies life and puts everything in perspective. Find the comic section in the newspaper or something funny to read and laugh. If someone is upset, try to analyze the situation from that person's perspective. Make yourself physically smile and laugh, it opens the blood vessels in the back of your head and physically lifts your mood. Choose to be happy in spite of circumstances. No one "makes" you happy – it's an attitude from within.

Thousands of people every year pay thousands of dollars for state-of-the-art testing to learn their risk for heart disease. However, experts say that fresh vegetables and fruits and a health club membership may be better buys than any lab test. People who eat a diet low in fat and cholesterol and rich in healthy plant foods, who don't smoke, who exercise regularly, and keep their weight and blood pressure in the normal range are less likely to have a heart attack than those who don't, despite any predisposition or genetic tendency toward heart disease. – Harvard Health Letter

Exercise is good for your health, but like everything else, it can be overdone. Too much exercise hampers the immune system. Couch potatoes need to exercise 30 minutes every day, but those who run, do high-impact aerobics or lift weights, need to take time off for the body to recharge and rest. A day of rest refuels your energy and motivation. Studies show that athletes who take a rest day occasionally, like once or twice a week, actually improved their performance over those who trained every day. – Shape Magazine

Juice Fasting – Introductory Road to Water Fasting

Fasting has been rediscovered through juice fasting as a simply delicious and easy means of cleansing and purifying and rebuilding health and vitality.

To fast (abstain from food) comes from the Old English word *fasten or to hold firm*. It's a means to commit oneself to the task of finding inner strength through cleansing of the body, mind and soul. Throughout history the world's greatest philosophers and sages – including Socrates, Plato, Buddha and Gandhi – have enjoyed fasting and preached its benefits.

Juice bars are springing up everywhere and juice fasting has become "in" with the Stars of Hollywood. The number of Stars who believe in the power and effectiveness of juice and water fasting is growing. Some are: Steven Spielberg, Barbara Streisand, Kim Basinger, Alec Baldwin, Christie Brinkley, Dolly Parton, Donna Karan, etc., and author Danielle Steel. They say fasting helps balance their lives physically, mentally, spiritually and emotionally.

Although a pure water fast is best, an introductory liquid juice fast can offer people an opportunity to give their intestinal systems restful, cleansing relief from the commercial, high-fat, sugar, salt, protein and "fast foods" diets that too many Americans exist on daily.

Organic raw live fruit and vegetable juices can be purchased fresh from many Health Stores. You can also prepare these healthy juices yourself using a good home juicer. When juice fasting, it's best to dilute the juice with ⅓ distilled water. This list gives you many delicious varieties. With vegetable and tomato combinations try adding a dash of Bragg Liquid Aminos or herbs. Non-fast days, try some of the nutritious green powders (barley, chlorella, spirulina, etc.) to create a powerful health drink. When using herbs in these drinks, use 1 to 2 fresh leaves or a pinch of dried herbs. A pinch of Dulse (seaweed) – rich in protein, iodine and iron – is delicious with vegetable juices.

Dine with little, sup with less; do better still, sleep supperless. – Ben Franklin

Paul C. Bragg Introduced Juicing to America

Juicing has come a long way since my father imported the first hand operated vegetable-fruit juicer from Germany. Before, this juice was pressed by hand using cheesecloth. He introduced his new juice therapy idea, then pineapple juice, then later tomato juice, to the American public. These two juices were erroneously thought to be too acid. Now, these health beverages have become the favorites of millions worldwide.

These are Some Powerful Juice Combinations:

1. Beet, celery, alfalfa sprouts
2. Cabbage, celery and apple
3. Cabbage, cucumber, celery, tomato, spinach and basil
4. Tomato, carrot and mint
5. Carrot, celery, watercress, garlic and wheatgrass
6. Grapefruit, orange and lemon
7. Beet, parsley, celery, carrot, mustard greens, cabbage, garlic
8. Beet, celery, dulse and carrot
9. Cucumber, carrot and parsley
10. Watercress, cucumber, garlic
11. Asparagus, carrot, and mint
12. Carrot, celery, parsley and cabbage, onion, sweet basil
13. Carrot and coconut milk
14. Carrot, broccoli, lemon, cayenne
15. Carrot, cauliflower, rosemary
16. Apple, carrot, radish, ginger
17. Apple, pineapple and mint
18. Apple, papaya and grapes
19. Papaya, cranberries and apple
20. Leafy greens, broccoli, apple
21. Grape, cherry and apple
22. Watermelon

99

Part of health success is preparation of purpose and goals.

Through our actions and deeds, rather than promises, let us display the essence of love – perfect harmony in motion!
– Philip Glyn, Welsh Poet

Little deeds of kindness, little words of love,
Help to make earth happy, like the Heaven above.
– Julia A. F. Carney

I used to say, "I sure hope things will change."
Then I learned that the only way things are going to change for me is when I change! – Jim Rohn

We shall never know all the good that a simple smile can do.

Increasing your intake of fruits and vegetables can help you prevent heart disease, cancer, and other chronic diseases. Surveys show that those who increased their daily fruit and vegetable intake improved their health, vitality and feelings of well-being. – UC Berkeley Wellness Letter

KEEP BIOLOGICALLY HEALTHY & YOUTHFUL WITH EXERCISE & GOOD NUTRITION

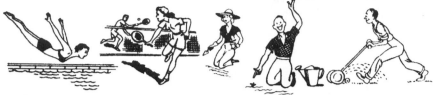

Always remember you have these vitally important reasons for following The Bragg Healthy Lifestyle:

- The ironclad laws of Mother Nature and God.
- Your common sense, which tells you that you are doing right.
- Your aim to make your health better and your life longer.
- Your resolve to prevent illness so that you may enjoy life.
- You will retain your faculties and be hale, hearty, active and useful far beyond the ordinary length of years.
- You will also possess superior mental and physical powers!
- By making an art of healthy living, you will be young at any age.

100

WANTED – For Robbing Health & Life

KILLER Saturated Fats	CHOKER Hydrogenated Fats
CLOGGER Salt	DEADEYED Devitalized Foods
DOPEY Caffeine	HARD Water (Inorganic Minerals)
PLUGGER Frying Pan	JERKY Turbulent Emotions
DEATH-DEALER Drugs	CRAZY Alcohol
GREASY Overweight	SMOKY Tobacco
HOGGY Over-eating	LOAFER Laziness

What Wise Men Say

Wisdom does not show itself so much in precept as in life – a firmness of mind and mastery of appetite. – Seneca

I saw few die of hunger – of eating, a hundred thousand.
– Ben Franklin

Govern well thy appetite, lest Sin surprise thee, and her black attendant, Death. – Milton

Health consists with temperance alone. – Pope

Our prayers should be for a sound mind in a healthy body. – Juvenal

Health is . . . a blessing that money cannot buy. – Izaak Walton

The natural healing force within us is the greatest force in getting well.
– Hippocrates, Father of Medicine

Of all the knowledge, that most worth having is knowledge about health! The first requisite of a good life is to be a healthy person. – Herbert Spencer

Chapter 10

Doctor Healthy Elimination – Mother Nature's Way

Banish Constipation Mother Nature's Way

Constipation is often referred to as the cause of many serious physical health problems. Yet few people know what a normal bowel movement means. The average person feels that if they have one bowel movement a day they are not constipated. This is not true! People who only have one daily bowel movement are chronically constipated and carry 5 to 10 pounds of putrefying, fermenting food material in their lower bowel. This produces irritation to the delicate lining of the bowel. The bowel then either tries to get rid of the irritations quickly – which results in diarrhea – or puts a spastic clamp on the intestines to keep them from producing further – resulting in constipation and other health problems.

Civilized people never seem to go to the root cause of their constipation – unhealthy lifestyle, lack of sufficient water (8 glasses of distilled water daily is important), no exercise and weak internal and external muscles of the abdomen. Americans spend over a billion dollars yearly trying to move their constipated bowels. But, all civilized countries sell large amounts of laxatives to move their cemented bowels.

The chief reason Americans need so much bowel "dynamite" is because they eat so much refined, mushy, lifeless, unnatural and empty-calorie foods. The refined grains and other foods have lost the B-complex vitamins needed to have a healthy and clean intestinal tract. Their digestive tract will lack tone unless vitamin B1 is present. Most diets consist of too many over-cooked, mushy foods that lack the tough cellulose fibers of raw vegetables that act as helpful, tiny intestinal brooms to give mobility, bulk, moisture and lubrication to the colon.

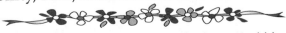

Good elimination is important for Super Health!

101

Raw Fresh Vegetables and Fruits Promote Healthy Elimination

The Bragg Healthy Lifestyle emphasizes at all times that a person should have 1 to 2 raw coarse salads a day. The base of these salads should be raw chopped or grated cabbage, carrots, beets, broccoli, cauliflower and celery. (Please see page 115 for our famous Bragg Healthy Salad Recipe!) The fleshy part of raw vegetables and fruits, contain cellulose, a colloidal element that retains water and acts as a soft bulk throughout the entire digestive system and helps promote good elimination!

If you cannot eat or tolerate coarser raw foods, then enjoy this tea after meals. Presoak enough flaxseed for several days (3 Tbsp to 1 pint distilled water). Store in glass jar. Add 1 Tbsp mixture to hot distilled water, juice or herbal tea and add ½ tsp psyllium husk powder. If desired add ½ tsp honey. Stir well and enjoy. This drink is a great bowel regulator and also rich in omega 3 and 6 oils.

Another suggestion for relieving constipation is to mix 1 tablespoon of crude blackstrap molasses in a cup of hot distilled water (it's also a healthy coffee substitute). You may also add ½ teaspoon psyllium husk powder to this drink. Have a cup upon arising and one an hour after dinner.

For easier-flowing, healthful bowel movements:

Squatting is the natural way to have a bowel movement. It opens up the anal area more directly. When on the toilet, putting your feet up 6 to 8 inches on a waste basket or footstool gives you the same squatting effect. If needed use your fingers behind to gently pull up on the edge of anus opening – this helps waste roll out easier!

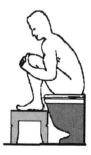

The body, soul and mind are so closely connected that not even a single word or thought can come into existence without being reflected in the personality and health of the individual. – John Prentiss

---

Eliminate the "dribbles": This will help keep the bladder and sphincter muscles tightened and toned: urinate – stop – urinate – stop, 6 times, twice daily when voiding. This simple exercise works. After age 40, do this every day.

Dream big, think big, but enjoy the small miracles of everyday life.

B-Complex Vitamins are Important for Intestinal Health and the Nervous System

The muscles of the intestinal tract may become flabby and prolapsed if the B-complex vitamins (especially B1) are not abundant in the diet. These water-soluble vitamins are not stored, but are lost in perspiration and urine, so be sure to include in your diet plenty of foods that are rich in the B vitamins. These foods include: raw wheat germ, brewer's yeast, blackstrap molasses, rice polishings, brown rice, barley, millet, quinoa, soybeans, dried peas and beans, cornmeal, buckwheat groats, mushrooms, broccoli, turnip and mustard greens, spinach, cabbage, peas, cantaloupe, grapefruit and oranges. It's also found in fish, beef steak, beef heart, lamb kidney and egg yolks – although we prefer the heart-healthy vegetarian sources.

Caution! Never, under any circumstances, use mineral oil as a laxative! It robs the body of the fat-soluble vitamins (A, D, E and K) that are waiting to be assimilated by the intestinal tract. Avoid all mineral oil products.

Preferably don't use enemas or colonic irrigations except in cases of sickness when there is a bowel blockage. Your nerves move your bowels. They can and will do the job if your vitamin B-complex intake is adequate and if your diet is correctly balanced with sufficient fiber (raw salads, vegetables, fruits, etc.), moisture, natural lubrication and 8 glasses of distilled water daily!

Keeping Clean Internally is the Secret To Health, Youthfulness and Long Life!

You should have a bowel movement on arising and 1 within an hour after each meal. Output must equal intake! Make it a practice to go to the toilet within 20 to 30 minutes after a meal and concentrate your entire mind on having a bowel evacuation. Use this squatting like position seen on page 102. It helps the abdominal muscles relax and open up normally, aiding in a more complete bowel movement. You should make a 10 minute effort to move the bowels after each meal.

8 Glasses of Water Daily Promotes Super Health and Healthy Elimination!

Cleanliness of the colon is important for superior health. If you are troubled by tenderness, soreness or hemorrhaging of the rectum, a peeled garlic bud – oiled, inserted as a suppository and allowed to remain overnight – has been found to be healing.

See that your daily liquid intake is at least 8 glasses of distilled water, plus some vegetable or fruit juice, especially if your bowel movements are dry. Many people suffer from constipation due to dehydration because they don't drink enough water. Remember salt, tea, coffee, alcohol, cola and soft drinks are dehydrating. One of the functions of the lower bowel is to remove surplus water from the waste. If wastes are not evacuated or remain in the colon too long and a great deal of water is removed, then the stools become too hard to easily eliminate. This painful condition can even damage delicate colon membranes causing hemorrhoids.

There is nothing as important to your health as good bowel elimination! Take care of this important function after each meal before too much of the liquid has been absorbed! Don't say that you are too busy. Bowel elimination is vital to vigorous health. These poisons must be moved out of the body – no meal should stay in the human colon more than 36 hours. We have trained our bowels to move a meal out of our bodies in 16 to 18 hours, and never more than 24 hours. When the normal rhythm of bowel evacuation is reached, many of your physical problems will vanish!

Terminator Sterile Seeds Threaten Food Freedom!

Terminator seeds are sterile crop seeds patented and marketed by the Monsanto Corp. that have been biologically altered to sprout a permanently infertile plant. The large scale use of these seeds (which is already underway in over 78 countries) could directly threaten the well-being of 1.4 billion people who now depend on food grown with fertile seeds. This would present a huge risk to the world because it could spread and sterilize all living plants, trees, etc. Farmers (and their neighbors, with plants 'accidently' cross-pollinated by Terminator plants) would be forced to buy new seeds every year. For many of these farmers financial ruin would result and bring on misery and famine for millions worldwide. Monsanto's seed program has no benefits for the world – only for the company's pocketbook. Discover Monsanto's fiendish plot to control the world's seed industry. Websites: rafi.org and sedos.org/Food/terminator.html

Famous Doctor Julian Whitaker Says:
Do as I Do – Drink Bragg's Apple Cider Vinegar

Julian Whitaker, M.D. and editor of the popular *HEALTH & HEALING* newsletter, writes that all vinegar is not created equal. He says that comparing organic, raw apple cider vinegar to distilled or synthetic vinegar is like comparing fresh-squeezed orange juice to Kool-Aid. "Do as I do," says Dr. Whitaker. "Drink warm water with a teaspoon each of Bragg's Organic Apple Cider Vinegar and raw honey every day!" This popular health newsletter feature also shared the following testimonials:

John R., a 76-year-old suffered from stomach distress his entire life. After $2,000 worth of medical tests, doctors recommended he take Zantac daily. A friend of John's had read about the healing qualities of apple cider vinegar and suggested he try it. John reports that his digestive problems disappeared after only one week of taking a daily dose of organic raw apple cider vinegar with honey in a glass of warm water. (Read page 114.)

105

Bob D., a 66-year-old patient being treated for heart disease, credits his twice daily "vinegar cocktails" for his rapid and remarkable elimination of angina pain, along with some other therapies. See web: drwhitaker.com

How to Improve Your Digestion

Millions have indigestion which is aggravated by poor digestion and weak saliva juices and causes indigestion: gas, heartburn and stomach bloating. Five minutes before mealtime, take 1 Tbsp. distilled water with ⅓ tsp. ACV. Before swallowing, hold in the mouth for a few seconds. This promotes saliva, which allows digestion to begin in the mouth. This small amount of diluted ACV causes stomach digestive fluids to flow faster, better and results in improved digestion.

Never chew gum! Chewing gum fools the body into thinking you are eating food and triggers the precious digestive juices to flow. This also promotes hunger. These strong juices cause trouble with your empty stomach's lining, resulting in stomach problems, bloating, ulcers, gas.

Foods Naturally Rich in Vitamin E

Here is a list of foods that contain the following notable amounts of precious vital vitamin E for your entire body and heart health. Compiled in *Bridges Food and Beverage Analyses*.

Food	Quantity	Vitamin E IU's
Apples	1 medium	0.74
Bananas	1 medium	0.40
Barley	½ cup	4.20
Beans, Navy	½ cup	3.60
Beef Steak	1 average piece	0.63
Beef Liver	1 average piece	1.40
Butter (salt-free)	6 tablespoons	2.40
Carrots	1 cup	0.45
Celery, Green	½ cup	2.60
Chicken	3 slices	0.25
Corn, Dried for Popcorn	1 cup	20.00
Cornmeal, Yellow	½ cup	1.70
Corn Oil	6 tablespoons	87.00
Eggs, Fertile	2	2.00
Endive, Escarole	½ cup	2.00
Flour, Whole Grain	1 cup	54.00
Grapefruit	½	0.52
Haddock	1 average piece	0.39
Kale	½ cup	8.00
Lamb Chops	2 rib chops	0.77
Lettuce	6 leaves	0.50
Mackerel, canned	½ cup	205.00
Oatmeal	½ cup	2.00
Olive Oil (Virgin)	½ cup	5.00
Onions, raw	2 medium	0.26
Oranges	1 small	0.24
Parsley	½ cup	5.50
Peas, Green	1 cup	4.00
Potatoes, White	1 medium	0.06
Potatoes, Sweet	1 small	4.00
Rice, Brown	¾ cup cooked	2.40
Rye	½ cup	3.00
Soybean Oil	6 tablespoons	140.00
Sunflower Seeds, raw	½ cup	31.00
Wheatgerm Oil	6 tablespoons	50-420.00

There's 54 Healthy Salad Recipes & 23 Delicious Dressing Recipes in the 448 page Bragg *Health Recipes Book*.

Chapter 11

Healthy Foods for a Youthful Body

Healthy High Vibration Foods Contain Life-Giving, Energy Substances

When you eat only foods that are in a high vibration, your body performs and operates by God's Universal Law. It becomes a self-starting, self-cleansing, self-governing, self-generating instrument! We want you to live by Mother Nature's and God's Laws so your body will be a fine working instrument at every age. If you desire to retain the vivaciousness, vitality, energy and enthusiasm of youth . . . if you have the desire to turn back the clock of Father Time when your body is tired and your gait is halting at an age when you should be buoyant with the spirit of youthfulness, then we say: *"There is but one healthy way to live and that is according to Mother Nature's and God's Eternal Laws!"*

BAD NUTRITION
#1 Cause of Sickness

People don't die of infectious conditions as such, but of malnutrition that allows the germs to gain a foothold in sickly bodies. Bad nutrition is usually one of the main causes of noninfectious, degenerative or fatal conditions. When the body has its full vitamin and mineral quota plus precious

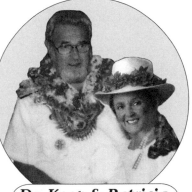

Dr. Koop & Patricia

potassium, it's impossible for germs to get a foothold in its healthy bloodstream and tissues! We greatly admire our friend, the former U.S. Surgeon General Dr. C. Everett Koop who, in his famous 1988 landmark report on nutrition and health, made this strong statement:

Diet-related diseases account for 68% of all United States deaths!

Apples are Powerful Nutritional Foods

"An apple a day keeps the doctor away," is a familiar saying known to millions. It carries truth and good common sense, because the apple is one of God's great health-giving foods.

Apples are a rich source of potassium, as vital to the soft tissues of the body as calcium is to the bones and harder tissues. Potassium is the mineral of youthfulness; it is the "artery softener," keeping the arteries of the body flexible and resilient. It is a fighter of dangerous bacteria and viruses. Yes, when you say, "An apple a day keeps the doctor away," you are talking good, down-to-earth old fashioned folk medicine for vibrant health!

The apple has stood the test of time. It is one of the oldest known fruits that humans consume. From the time of the Garden of Eden the apple has played a vital part in our destiny. People have been eating apples for thousands of years. Apple eaters enjoy a certain healthfulness that non-apple eaters never achieve.

Fight Arthritis with Apple Cider Vinegar

Hard, stony deposits fill up, cement, enlarge and cripple the joints! Crippling, painful arthritis and joint problems are the sad result! Fight and help flush out those stony deposits with Apple Cider Vinegar and by being faithful to The Bragg Healthy Lifestyle. Eat 60% to 70% healthy raw foods (organic is best), drink 8 glasses of pure distilled water (free of chemicals and inorganic minerals) and take your multi vitamin-mineral supplements, kelp and alfalfa tablets and 1 tsp. cod liver oil daily. You will be amazed by the great health improvements!

Upon arising, an hour before lunch and dinner have your delicious ACV cocktail as follows: Stir 6 ounces distilled water with 1 to 2 tsp. equally of ACV and (optional) raw honey. Also, sprinkle ACV over your daily garden salads and steamed greens. Remember, eating 1 to 2 organic apples a day helps keep the doctor and his bills away!

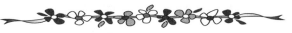

Remember, you are punished by your bad habits of living. – Paul C. Bragg

Keep Your Joints and Tissues Youthful

Most people have lost their normal contact with Mother Nature and simple, natural living. They no longer know how to eat the simple way God intended.

If you suffer from prematurely old joints and hardened tissues, take the ACV mixture three times daily. Eliminate or cut down on animal proteins. Stop using all refined sugars, products and beverages! Then you will soon see how very youthful your body will begin to feel.

After several months on the Bragg Healthy Lifestyle and the ACV and honey cocktail taken 3 times daily, you will find that joint stiffness and misery starts vanishing. You will discover you can walk or run up stairs without effort! You will notice that you look younger and feel younger than you have in years! (Also, follow page 121.)

Make The Bragg Healthy Lifestyle a life-long daily habit! Over the years we have seen many stiff-jointed, prematurely old people transform themselves into new, youthful, healthy people! We cannot do it for you. You must make the effort to give this ACV and honey program a chance to prove what it can do for you! Don't procrastinate: we challenge you to begin today!

109

Your Waistline is Your Life-Line, Date-Line and Health-Line!

Get a tape measure and measure your waist. Write down the measurement. If you consciously pursue vigorous abdominal and postural exercises combined with correct eating and a weekly 24 hour fast (and, later on, 3 to 7 day fasts), in a short time you'll see a more trim and youthful waistline. Trim waistlines can make people appear years younger. Now, let's get yours down to where it should be, if it has grown too big and fat. It's a trim, lean horse for the long race of life! I'm sure we all want longevity! Studies show the bigger the waistline – the shorter the lifespan. Living The Bragg Healthy Lifestyle is so wonderful. Each day is a precious gift to enjoy, treasure and guard . . . for the healthy life is truly wonderful and beautiful and so rewarding!

Most People Abuse Their Stomachs

People abuse their stomachs! You can't overeat dead, empty-calorie foods night and day and tell yourself that it won't harm or show on you! You are completely wrong! Devitalized foods create toxic poisons inside your body and add unhealthy, flabby inches to your stomach and body. Don't overeat even healthy foods, for your body only needs enough food (fuel) to maintain energy. When you see fat people, it's because they have stuffed too much food into their bodies. Flesh is dumb.

Have you over-fueled your body? If so, you are not getting away with this harmful habit, you are abusing your health and cheating yourself! Keep in mind that as we live longer, the internal abdominal structure and stomach muscles relax more. This is called visceroptosis, or droopy tummy. It's a common condition among older people who overeat and don't exercise their waist muscles. It can be a contributing cause of constipation, body sluggishness, prolapsed liver and even hernias.

When the abdominal wall becomes lazy, the droop is compounded by fat layers of flab, then trouble starts inside the abdomen. Most people by 40 have a prolapsed abdomen. Become a people-watcher and you will notice this is true! Some need a surgical tummy-tuck (removes excess flab) to give them a flat stomach. So, don't let your abdominal muscles droop! Make every effort to recapture firmness. It's amazing how quickly muscles respond to good posture and simple, easy-to-do exercises.

The Bragg Posture Exercise

Tighten the butt, suck in stomach muscles, lift up ribcage and stretch up the spine. Keep the chest up and out, shoulders back and lift the chin up slightly and line the spine up straight (nose plumbline straight to belly button). Drop the hands to the sides and swing them to normalize your posture. Do this exercise before a mirror and see miraculous changes. You are retraining and strengthening your muscles to sit, stand and walk tall and straight for more youthfulness and health!

WHERE DO YOU STAND?

POSTURE CHART

	PERFECT	FAIR	POOR
HEAD			
SHOULDERS			
SPINE			
HIPS			
ANKLES			
NECK			
UPPER BACK			
TRUNK			
ABDOMEN			
LOWER BACK			

111

From your head to your feet, your posture carries you through life.
This is your human vehicle and you are truly a miracle! Cherish, respect
and protect it by living The Bragg Healthy Lifestyle. – Patricia Bragg

Your posture can make or break your health!

Foods and Allergies

Every known food may cause some allergic reaction at times. Thus the foods used in "elimination" diets may cause allergic reactions in some individuals and a few are listed among the "Most Common Food Allergies." Since the incidence of reaction to these foods is generally low, they are widely used in making test diets. By keeping your own food journal you will soon know your "problem" foods that must be eliminated from your diet.

After eating some particular type of food, especially if it happens each time you eat that food, your body has a reaction, the chances are you may have an allergy. Here are some of the allergic reactions and they can happen very quickly! You might wheeze, sneeze, develop a stuffy nose, nasal drip or mucus, dark circles or waterbags under your eyes, headaches, feel light-headed or dizzy, heart beats faster, stomach and chest pains, diarrhea, extreme thirst, break out in a rash or have a swelling of the tissues (ankles, feet, hands or stomach bloating, etc.) either externally or internally.

If you know what you're allergic to, you are lucky; if you don't, you had better find out as fast as possible and eliminate all irritating foods from your diet. To re-evaluate your daily life and have a guide to your future start a daily journal (8½ x 11 notebook) of foods eaten and your reactions, moods, energy levels, weight, elimination and sleep patterns. Soon you will discover the foods and situations causing problems. By charting your diet you will be amazed at the effects of eating certain foods. Paul C. Bragg faithfully kept his journal for over 70 years.

112

If you are hypersensitive to certain foods, you must reject them from your diet! There are hundreds of allergies and of course it is impossible here to take up each one. Many who suffer from this unpleasant affliction have allergies to wheat, milk or eggs, while some persons are allergic to all grains. Your journal will help you discover and accurately pinpoint the foods and situations causing your problems. Start today!

Most Common Food Allergies to Check For:

- *MILK: Butter, Cheese, Cottage Cheese, Ice Cream, Milk, Yogurt, etc.*
- *CEREALS & GRAINS: Wheat, Corn, Buckwheat, Oats, Rye*
- *EGGS: Cakes, Custards, Dressings, Mayonnaise, Noodles*
- *FISH: Shellfish, Crab, Lobster, Shrimp, Shadroe*
- *MEATS: Bacon, Chicken, Pork, Sausage, Veal, Smoked Products*
- *FRUITS: Citrus Fruits, Melons, Strawberries* **
- *VEGETABLES: Brussels Sprouts, Cauliflower, Celery, Eggplant, Legumes, Onions, Potatoes, Spinach, Tomatoes*
- *NUTS: Peanuts, Pecans, Walnuts, all chemically dried and preserved*
- *MISCELLANEOUS: Chocolate, China Tea, Cocoa, Coffee, MSG, Palm and Cottonseed Oils, Salt, Spices.* * *Allergic reactions are often from toxic pesticides on salad greens, vegetables, fruits, etc.*

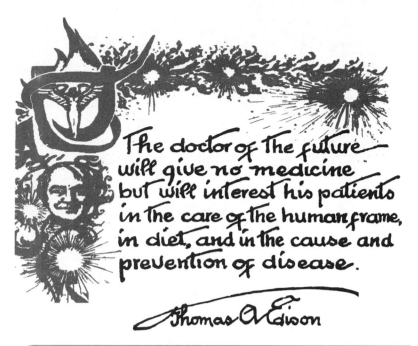

The doctor of the future will give no medicine but will interest his patients in the care of the human frame, in diet, and in the cause and prevention of disease.

Thomas A. Edison

Enjoy Healthy Fiber for Super Health

- KEEP BEANS HANDY, probably the best fiber sources. Cook dried beans and freeze in portions. Use canned beans for faster meals.

- EAT BERRIES, surprisingly good sources of fiber.

- INSTEAD OF ICEBERG LETTUCE, choose deep green lettuces, romaine, bib, butter, etc., spinach or cabbage for variety salads.

- LOOK FOR "100% WHOLE WHEAT" or whole grain breads. A dark color isn't proof; check labels, compare fibers, grains, etc.

- WHOLE GRAIN CEREALS. Hot, also cold granolas with sliced fruit.

- GO FOR BROWN RICE. It's better for you and so delicious.

- EAT THE SKINS of potatoes and other organic fruits and vegetables.

- LOOK FOR HEALTH CRACKERS with at least 2 grams of fiber per ounce.

- SERVE HUMMUS, made from chickpeas, instead of sour-cream dips.

- USE WHOLE WHEAT FLOUR for baking breads, muffins, pastries, pancakes, waffles and for variety try other whole grain flours.

- DON'T UNDERESTIMATE CORN, including popcorn, corn tortillas.

- ADD OAT BRAN, WHEAT BRAN AND WHEATGERM to baked goods, cookies, etc.; whole grain cereals, casseroles, loafs, etc.

- SNACK ON SUN-DRIED FRUIT, such as apricots, dates, prunes, raisins, etc., which are concentrated sources of nutrients and fiber.

- INSTEAD OF DRINKING JUICE, eat the fruit: orange, grapefruit, etc.; and vegetables: tomato, carrot, etc. – UC Berkeley Wellness Letter

Healthy organic foods have a wonderful abundance of potential life energy.

These freshly squeezed organic vegetable and fruit juices are important to The Bragg Healthy Lifestyle. It's not wise to drink beverages with your main meals, as it dilutes the digestive juices. But it's great during the day to have a glass of freshly squeezed orange, grapefruit, vegetable juice, Bragg Vinegar Drink, herb tea or try a hot cup of Bragg Liquid Aminos Broth (½ to 1 tsp Bragg Liquid Aminos in cup of hot distilled water) – these are all ideal pick-me-up beverages.

Bragg Apple Cider Vinegar Cocktail – Mix 1 to 2 tsps equally Bragg Organic ACV and (optional) raw honey in 8 oz. of distilled water. Take 1 glass upon arising, an hour before lunch and dinner. Read page 116.

Delicious Hot Cider Health Drink – Add 2 cinnamon sticks and cloves to hot distilled water, steep for 20 minutes. Before drinking add Bragg Raw Organic Apple Cider Vinegar and raw honey to your taste.

Bragg Favorite Juice Cocktail – This drink consists of all raw vegetables (please remember organic is best) which we prepare in our vegetable juicer: carrots, celery, beets, cabbage, watercress and parsley. The great purifier, fresh garlic we enjoy, but it's optional.

Bragg Healthy "Pep" Drink – After our morning stretch and exercises we often enjoy this instead of fruit. It's also delicious and powerfully nutritious as a meal anytime: lunch, dinner or take along in a thermos to work, school, the gym, or to the park or hiking, etc.

Bragg Healthy Pep Drink

Prepare following in blender, add (distilled water) ice cube if desired:
Juice of: freshly squeezed orange, grapefruit or tangelo; or carrot & greens; or unsweetened pineapple; or 1½ cups distilled water with:

1 to 2 bananas, ripe	*⅓ tsp nutritional yeast flakes*
⅓ tsp flaxseed oil, optional	*1 tsp raw honey, optional*
½ tsp green powder (barley, etc.)	*½ tsp lecithin granules*
½ tsp psyllium husk powder	*1 tsp soy protein powder*
½ tsp raw oat bran	*⅓ tsp vitamin C powder*
1 tsp raw sunflower seeds	*½ tsp raw wheat germ*

Optional: 4 apricots (sun dried, unsulphured). Soak in jar overnight in distilled water or unsweetened pineapple juice. We soak enough to last for several days. Keep refrigerated. In summer, you can add fresh fruit in season: peaches, strawberries, berries, apricots, etc. instead of the banana. In winter, add apples, kiwi, oranges, pears or persimmons or try sugar-free, frozen organic fruits. Serves 1 to 2.

Patricia's Delicious Health Popcorn

Use freshly popped popcorn (I prefer air popped). If desired, use olive, soy, sesame or flax seed oil. Add pinch of Italian or French herbs, cayenne pepper, mustard powder or fresh crushed garlic to oil. Pour the oil over popcorn and then add several sprays of Bragg Liquid Aminos and Bragg Organic Apple Cider Vinegar. Sprinkle with nutritional yeast large flakes (rich in B-complex). Try – delicious served instead of bread.

Bragg Lentil & Brown Rice Casserole

14 oz pkg lentils, uncooked
4 carrots, chop
3 celery stalks, chop
2 onions, chop
4 garlic cloves, chop

1 cup organic brown, rice, uncooked
3 quarts distilled water
1 tsp Bragg Liquid Aminos
½ tsp Italian herbs (oregano, basil, etc.)
2 tsp olive oil (virgin - first press is best)

Wash & drain lentils and rice. Place grains in large stainless steel pot. Add water. Bring to boil, reduce heat, simmer for 30 minutes. Then add vegetables & seasonings to rice & cook on low heat until done. Just before serving, add fresh or canned tomatoes. For a delicious garnish add parsley & nutritional yeast (large) flakes. Add more water in cooking the grains to make a delicious soup or stew. Serves 4 to 6.

Bragg Raw Vegetable Health Salad

2 stalks celery, chop
1 bell pepper & seeds, dice
½ cucumber, unwaxed, chop
1 carrot, grate
1 raw beet, grate
1 cup green cabbage, slice

½ cup red cabbage, chop
½ cup alfalfa or sunflower sprouts
2 spring onions & tops, chop
1 turnip, grate
1 avocado (ripe)
3 tomatoes, medium size

Chop, slice or grate vegetables fine to medium for variety in size. For variety add raw zucchini, sugar peas, mushrooms, broccoli, cauliflower. Mix vegetables thoroughly & serve on a bed of lettuce, spinach, watercress or chopped cabbage. Dice avocado & tomato and serve on side as a dressing. Serve choice of fresh squeezed lemon, orange or dressing separately. Chill salad plates before serving. Always eat your raw health salad first before serving hot dishes. Serves 3 to 5.

Bragg Vinaigrette Health Dressing

½ cup Bragg Apple Cider Vinegar
2 tsps raw honey
⅓ tsp Bragg Liquid Aminos
1 to 2 cloves garlic, minced
⅓ cup virgin olive oil or blend with safflower, sesame. soy or flax oil
1 Tbsp fresh herbs, minced or a pinch of Italian or French dry herbs

Blend ingredients in blender or jar. Refrigerate in covered jar.

For delicious herbal vinegar: in quart jar add ⅓ cup tightly packed, crushed fresh sweet basil, tarragon, dill, oregano, or any fresh herbs desired, combined or singly. (If *dried* herbs, use 1 to 2 tsp. herbs.) Now cover to top with Bragg Organic Raw Apple Cider Vinegar and store in warm place for two weeks, then strain and refrigerate.

Honey – Celery Seed Vinaigrette

¼ tsp dry mustard
¼ tsp Bragg Liquid Aminos
¼ tsp paprika
3 Tbsp raw honey

1 cup Bragg Apple Cider Vinegar
½ cup virgin olive oil
Pinch of salad herbs
⅓ tsp celery seed

Blend ingredients in blender or jar. Refrigerate in covered jar.

You are what you eat, drink, breathe, think and do! – Patricia Bragg

THE MIRACLES OF APPLE CIDER VINEGAR FOR A STRONGER, LONGER, HEALTHIER LIFE

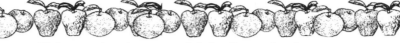

The old adage is true:
"An apple a day helps keep the doctor away."

- Helps maintain a youthful, vibrant body
- Helps fight germs and bacteria naturally
- Helps retard the onset of old age in humans, pets and farm animals
- Helps regulate calcium metabolism
- Helps keep blood the right consistency
- Helps regulate women's menstruation
- Helps normalize the urine, thus relieving the frequent urge to urinate
- Helps digestion and assimilation
- Helps relieve sore throats, laryngitis and throat tickles and cleans out toxins
- Helps sinus, asthma and flu sufferers to breathe easier and more normally
- Helps maintain healthy skin, soothes sunburn
- Helps prevent itching scalp, dry hair and baldness, and banishes dandruff
- Helps fight arthritis and removes crystals and toxins from joints, tissues and organs
- Helps control and normalize weight

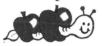

– Paul C. Bragg, Health Crusader, Originator of Health Stores

Our sincere blessings to you, dear friends, who make our lives so worthwhile and fulfilled by reading our teachings on natural living as our Creator laid down for us to follow. He wants us to follow the simple path of natural living. This is what we teach in our books and health crusades worldwide. Our prayers reach out to you and your loved ones for the best in health and happiness. We must follow the laws He has laid down for us, so we can reap this precious health physically, mentally, emotionally and spiritually!

With Love,

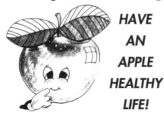

HAVE AN APPLE HEALTHY LIFE!

Braggs Organic Raw Apple Cider Vinegar with the "Mother" is the #1 food I recommend to maintain the body's vital acid – alkaline balance.
– Gabriel Cousens, M.D., Author, *Conscious Eating*

Food and Product Summary

Today, many of our foods are highly processed or refined, which robs them of essential nutrients, vitamins, minerals and enzymes. Many also contain harmful and dangerous chemicals. The research findings and experience of top scientists, physicians, dentists and nutritionists have led to the discovery that devitalized foods are major causes of poor health, illness, cancer and premature death. The enormous increase in the last 70 years of degenerative diseases such as heart disease, arthritis and dental decay substantiate this belief. Scientific research shows that most of these afflictions can be prevented and that others, once established, may be arrested or even reversed through nutritional methods.

Enjoy Super Health with Natural Foods

1. **RAW FOODS:** Use fresh fruits and raw vegetables; the organically grown are always best. Enjoy nutritious variety garden salads with sprouts and raw nuts and seeds.

2. **VEGETABLE and ANIMAL PROTEINS:**
   a. Legumes, lentils, brown rice, soybeans and beans.
   b. Nuts and seeds, raw and unsalted.
   c. Animal protein (if you must), hormone free, organic meats, liver, kidney, brain, heart, poultry, seafood. Please eat these proteins sparingly or it's best to enjoy the healthier vegetarian diet. You can bake, roast, wok or broil these proteins. Eat meat no more than 3 times a week.
   d. Dairy products – eggs (fertile, free range), unprocessed hard cheese, goat's cheese and certified raw milk. We choose not to use dairy products. Try the healthier soy, nut (almond, etc.) and Rice Dream – the non-dairy milks.

3. **FRUITS and VEGETABLES:** When possible organic is best because it's grown without the use of poisonous sprays and toxic chemical fertilizers. Ask your market to stock organic produce. Steam, bake, sauté or wok veggies for as short a time as possible to retain the most nutritional content and flavor. Also enjoy fresh juices.

4. **100% WHOLE GRAIN CEREALS, BREADS and FLOURS:** They contain important B-complex vitamins, vitamin E, minerals and the important unsaturated fatty acids.

5. **COLD or EXPELLER-PRESSED VEGETABLE OILS:** Virgin olive oil, soy, sunflower, flax and sesame oils are excellent sources of healthy, essential, unsaturated fatty acids; but it's still wise to use all oils sparingly.

There is a great deal of truth in the saying that man becomes what he eats. – Gandhi

Pure Water is Important for Health

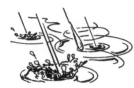

To the days of the aged it addeth length;
To the might of the strong it addeth strength;
It freshens the heart, it brings us delight;
'Tis like drinking a goblet of morning light.

The body is 70% water and pure, steam-distilled (chemical-free) water is important for total health. You should drink 7-9 glasses of water a day. Read our book, *Water – The Shocking Truth* for more information on the importance of pure water. See back pages for book list.

Pure distilled water is vitally important in following The Bragg Healthy Lifestyle. Water is the key to all body functions including: digestion, circulation, bones and joints, assimilation, elimination, muscles, nerves, glands and the senses. The right kind of water is one of your best natural protections against all kinds of diseases and viral infections, such as influenza and pneumonia. Water is vital factor in all body fluids, tissues, cells, lymph, blood and all glandular secretions. Water holds all nutritive factors in solution, as well as toxins and body wastes, and acts as the main transportation medium throughout the body for nutrition and cleansing purposes!

Low Fat Meals Cut Heart Disease Risk

A British research report by Dr. George Miller of Britain's Medical Research Council stated: *"High fat meals make the blood more prone to clot within 6 to 7 hours after eating. Low fat meals can almost immediately reverse this condition. Most heart attacks occur in the early morning. One reason may be the overnight clotting effects of a high fat dinner. Researchers feel that by cutting fats from your diet, you may be able to add years to your life and cut the risk of heart disease!"* Also, recent University of Chicago scientific research findings support Dr. Miller's strong statement that the safest heart healthy meals are the low fat, vegetarian diets with ample fruits and vegetables.

A wise man should consider that health is the greatest of human blessings!
– Hippocrates, Father of Medicine, 400 B.C.

Vegetables & Grains – Healthy Proteins

Many vegetables, grains and legumes are excellent protein sources (chart page 17), including soybeans, tofu, brown and wild rice, lima beans, garbanzos, split peas, lentils, pinto and kidney beans. All beans are good sources of protein and magnesium and are important for a healthy heart and also wise "health insurance"!

If you desire meat, *(hormone-free and drug-free)* *don't eat it more than 2-3 times weekly.* Meat has uric acid, urea, saturated fats and cholesterol. These are all toxic materials and not good for the body. If desired, substitute fish, chicken or turkey because these are cleaner proteins with less saturated fat, uric acid and urea than red meat. Free-range poultry is better for you than red meat. We prefer you learn to enjoy a heart-healthy vegetarian diet.

Eggs (free-range, fertile eggs are best) should not be eaten over 4 *times a week.* They are a highly concentrated food with cholesterol, a saturated fat, in the yolk. If your count is over 200, leave eggs out until your cholesterol gets to 180 or lower (see page 121). Milk cheeses are highly concentrated. If you eat cheese have naturally aged and feta (goat/sheep cheese) occasionally. Never eat processed cheese. Dairy products are mucus producing – eat them sparingly or not at all! Enjoy healthy soy cheeses instead.

119

Slowly start cutting down on an unbalanced, heavy, unhealthy breakfast; start including more fresh fruit, stewed prunes with raw wheat germ, honey and fresh fruit make a nutritious breakfast. In time, you can learn to eat lightly or not at all, for most people don't need breakfast. There aren't two people any more physically and mentally active than my father and I. We never eat breakfast, other than fresh fruit or the Bragg Healthy Pep Drink on page 114. Before we eat even that, we enjoy our morning exercises, practicing our deep breathing or taking a long hike or swim. Our day starts early and we are busy until 10 a.m. before we have our fruit. Many mornings, we are so busy writing books for you, our readers and friends, that we don't even take time to eat! We love being Health Crusaders and sharing with you!

People don't fail because they intended to;
they fail to do what they intended to do.

Most Americans Overeat!

Overeating robs energy! Don't overeat, even healthy foods! Help your body detoxify by giving it cleansing time! When you eat, your body is forced to work on digesting food and has no energy for detoxification. So in time the toxins and waste pile up and then you accumulate physical miseries and age prematurely. Don't over-burden your amazing human machinery and kill yourself prematurely! Life is precious and we want you alive, healthy and happy for a long life!

Diet related premature death is an unnecessary tragedy!

Warning! – Avoid All Unhealthy Microwaved Foods!

In the past 20 years microwaves have practically replaced traditional methods of cooking, especially with the on-the-go people of today's world. But how much do you really know about them? Are they no more than timesaving machines for cooking? A Swiss study found that food which is microwaved is not the food it was before. The microwave radiation deforms and destroys the molecular structure of the food - creating radiolytic compounds. When microwaved food is eaten, abnormal changes occur in the blood and immune systems. These include a decrease in hemoglobin and white blood cell counts and an increase in cholesterol levels. An article in the journal Pediatrics warns that microwaving human milk damages the anti-infective properties it usually gives to a mother's baby. Recent work being done at the University of Warwick in Great Britain warns that microwave radiation is damaging to the electromagnetic activity of human life vibrations. See info on website: warwick.ac.uk/news/pr/97. Over 20 years ago Russia established microwave radiation limits 1000 times more stringent than in the United States and Great Britan. See web: • 203.23.131/nexus/microwave.html • health.microworld.com/html/microwave.html

Old age is a highly toxic condition caused by nutritional deficiencies and an unhealthy lifestyle!

Aspartame – Artificial Diet Sweetener Unhealthy & Makes You Fat!

Because Monsanto's artificial sweetener aspartame (sold as "Nutrasweet," "Equal," and "Spoonful") is over 200 times sweeter than sugar, it's a common ingredient found in "diet" foods and has become a sweetening staple for dieters. Besides being a deadly poison (see page 42), aspartame actually contributes to weight gain by causing a craving for carbohydrates. A study of 80,000 women by the American Cancer Society found that those who used this neurotoxic "diet" sweetener actually gained more weight than those who didn't use aspartame products. Find out more about the deadly health risks posed by Monsanto's toxic sweetener on this website: aspartamekills.com. Stevia, a herbal sweetener is a healthy alternative.

Healthy Heart Habits for a Long, Vital Life

Remember, organic live foods make live people; you are what you eat, drink, breathe, think and do; so eat a low-fat, low-sugar, high-fiber diet of natural whole grains, sprouts, fresh salad greens, vegetables, fruits, raw seeds, nuts, juices and chemical-free, pure distilled water.

Earn your food with daily exercise, for regular exercise improves your health, stamina, flexibility and endurance, and helps open the cardiovascular system. Only 45 minutes a day can do miracles for your mind and body. You become revitalized with new zest for living.

We are made of tubes. To help keep them clean and open, make a mixture using equal parts raw oat bran and psyllium husk powder. Add 1 to 3 tsps daily to juices, pep drinks, herb teas, soups, hot cereals, foods, etc. Also I take 1 cayenne capsule (40,000 HU) daily with meals.

Another way to guard against clogged tubes daily is add 2 Tbsps soy lecithin granules (fat emulsifier) to beverages, veggies, soups, etc.

Take 50 to 100 mgs regular-released niacin (B-3) with one meal daily to help cleanse and open the cardiovascular system. Skin flushing may occur; don't worry about this as it shows it's working! After your cholesterol level reaches 180 or lower, take 2 to 3 niacin weekly.

The heart needs a healthy balance of nutrients, so take a natural multi-vitamin-mineral food supplement with extra natural vitamin E, vitamin C, magnesium orotate, MSM, selenium, zinc, beta carotene and the amino acid L-Carnitine–these are the heart's super helpers! It's also wise to take bromelain and a multi-digestive enzyme with each meal – it aids digestion, assimilation and elimination.

Sleep problems try melatonin, magnesium, calcium, Sleepytime herb tea.

For arthritis, osteoarthritis, pain & stiffness, try glucosamine & chondroitin, it helps heal & regenerate. Also try capsaicin & DMSO lotion.

Use amazing antioxidants – vitamin C, grape seed extract, SOD, selenium, etc. They improve the immune system and help flush out dangerous free radicals that cause havoc with the cardiovascular pipes and health. Research shows antioxidents promote longevity, slow ageing, fight toxins, help prevent cataracts, jet lag, exhaustion & disease.

Count your blessings daily while you do your 30 to 45 minute brisk walks and exercises with these affirmations – health! strength! youth! vitality! peace! laughter! humility! understanding! forgiveness! joy! and love for eternity!– and soon all these qualities will come flooding and bouncing into your life. With blessings of super health, peace and love to you, our dear friends – our readers. – Patricia Bragg

Recommended Blood Chemistry Values

- Total Cholesterol: 180 mg/dl or less; 150 mg/dl or less is optimal
- Total Cholesterol, Childhood Years: 140 mg/dl or less
- HDL Cholesterol: Men, 50 mg/dl or more; Women, 65 mg/dl or more
- HDL Cholesterol Ratio: 3.2 or less • Triglycerides: 100 mg/dl or less
- LDL Cholesterol: 100 mg/dl or less is optimal • Glucose: 80 -100 mg/dl

121

Exercises Help Keep You More Youthful, Healthier, Stronger, Flexible and Trim

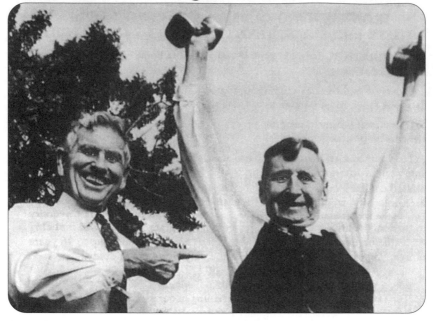

Paul C. Bragg and Friend, Roy White, 106 Years Young

They both practice progressive weight training 3 times a week for staying healthy and fit. Scientists have proven that weight training works miracles for all ages in maintaining flexibility, energy and youthful stamina!

Some amazing scientific data from around the world on important studies researching longevity and health report the renewing and rewarding benefits of regular exercise and living a healthy lifestyle!

Good health, generated by physical fitness is the logical starting point for the pursuit of excellence in any field. Physical vitality promotes mental vitality and thus is essential to executive achievement.
– Dr. Richard E, Dutton, University of Southern Florida

While exercise is important, cooling down afterward is just as essential. This includes about five minutes of less-intensive exercise similar to the activity just performed. This lowers your adrenaline level and helps keep blood from pooling in the legs. Adrenaline that remains in the bloodstream stresses the heart and pooling of blood lowers blood pressure suddenly and could cause a reduced blood flow to the heart and cause light-headedness. – Johns Hopkins Medical Letter

Chapter 12

Alternative Health Therapies And Massage Techniques

Try Them – They Work Miracles!

Explore these wonderful natural methods of healing your body. Then choose the techniques best for you:

Acupuncture/Acupressure – Acupuncture directs and rechannels body energy by inserting hair-thin needles (use only disposable needles) at specific points on the body. It's used for pain, backaches, migraines and general body dysfunction. Used in Asia for centuries, acupuncture is safe, virtually painless and has no side effects. Acupressure is based on the same principles and uses finger pressure and massage rather than needles. Websites offer info – check them out. Web: acupuncture.com

Chiropractic – Daniel David Palmer founded chiropractic in 1885 in Davenport, Iowa. There are now 16 schools in the U.S., and graduates are joining Health Practitioners in all the modern nations of the world to share healing techniques. Chiropractic is the largest healing profession and benefits millions. Treatment involves soft tissue, spinal and body adjustment to free the nervous system of interferences with normal body function. Its concern is the functional integrity of the musculoskeletal system. In addition to manual methods, chiropractors use physical therapy modalities, exercise, health and nutritional guidance. Web: chiropractic.org

123

F. Mathius Alexander Technique – Lessons to end improper use of neuromuscular system and bring body posture back into balance. Eliminates psycho-physical interferences, helps release long-held tension, and aids in re-establishing muscle tone. Web: alexandertechnique.com

Feldenkrais Method – Founded by Dr. Moshe Feldenkrais in the late 1940s. Lessons lead to improved posture and help create ease and efficiency of movement. A great stress removal method. Web: feldenkrais.com

No man can violate Nature's Laws and escape her penalties. – Julian Johnson

Homeopathy – Dr. Samuel Hahnemann developed homeopathy in the 1800s. Patients are treated with minute amounts of substances similar to those that cause a particular disease to trigger the body's own defenses. The homeopathic principle is *like cures like.* This safe and nontoxic remedy is the #1 alternative therapy in Europe and Britain because it is inexpensive, seldom has any side effects, and often brings fast results. Web: homeopthyhome.com

Naturopathy – Brought to America by Dr. Benedict Lust, M.D., this treatment uses diet, herbs, homeopathy, fasting, exercise, hydrotherapy, manipulation and sunlight. (Dr. Paul C. Bragg graduated from Dr. Lust's first School of Naturopathy in the U.S.) Practitioners work with your body to restore health naturally. They reject surgery and drugs except as a last resort. Web: naturopathics.com

Osteopathy – The first School of Osteopathy was founded in 1892 by Dr. Andrew Taylor Still, M.D. There are now 15 such colleges in the U.S. Treatment involves soft tissue, spinal and body adjustments that free the nervous system from interferences that can cause illness. Healing by adjustment also includes good nutrition, physical therapies, proper breathing and good posture. Dr. Still's premise was that structure and function of the human body are interdependent; if the body structure is altered or abnormal, function is altered and illness results. Web: osteopathy.com

124

Reflexology or Zone Therapy – Founded by Eunice Ingham, author of "The Story The Feet Can Tell," inspired by a Bragg Health Crusade when she was 17. Reflexology helps the body by removing crystalline deposits from meridians (nerve endings) of the feet through deep pressure massage. A form of Reflexology has its early origins in China and is known to have been practiced by Kenyan Natives and Native American Indian tribes for centuries. Reflexology helps activate the body's flow of healthy energy by dislodging any collected deposits. Web: reflexology.org

Skin Brushing is wonderful for circulation, toning, cleansing and healing. Use a dry vegetable brush (never nylon) and brush lightly. Removes old skin cells, uric acid crystals and toxic wastes that come up through the skin's pores. Try a loofah sponge for variety in the shower or tub.

Reiki – A Japanese form of massage that means "Universal Life Energy." Reiki helps the body to detoxify, then rebalance and heal itself. Discovered in the ancient Sutra manuscripts by Dr. Mikso Usui in 1822. Web: reiki.com

Rolfing – Developed by Ida Rolf in the 1930s in the U.S. Rolfing is also called structural processing and postural release or structural dynamics. It is based on the concept that distortions (accidents, injuries, falls, etc.) and the effects of gravity on the body cause upsets in the body. Rolfing helps to achieve balance and improved body posture. Methods involve the use of stretching, deep tissue massage and relaxation techniques to loosen old injuries and break bad movement and posture patterns, which can cause long-term health and body stress. Web: rolf.org

Tragering – Founded by Dr. Milton Trager M.D., who was inspired at age 18 by Paul C. Bragg to become a doctor. It is an experimental learning method that involves gentle shaking and rocking, suggesting a greater letting go, releasing tensions and lengthening of muscles for more body health. Tragering can do miraculous healing where needed in the muscles and the entire body. Web: trager.com

Water Therapy – For a great shower, apply almond, avocado, sesame or olive oil to skin, then alternate hot and cold water and massage needed areas while under spray. Garden hose massage is great in summer. Tub baths are wonderful, apply oil and massage. For muscle aches, add 1 cup apple cider vinegar or Epsom salts. Web:nmsnt.org

Massage & Aromatherapy – works two ways: the essence (smell) relaxes as does the massage. Essential oils are extracted from flowers, leaves, roots, seeds and barks. These are usually massaged into the skin, inhaled or used in a bath for their qualities to relax, soothe and heal. The oils, used for centuries to treat numerous ailments, are revitalizing and energizing for the body and mind. Example: Tiger Balm, echinacea and arnica help relieve muscle aches. Avoid skin creams and lotions with mineral oil because it clogs the skin's pores. Use these natural oils for the skin: almond, apricot kernel, avocado, soy, hemp seed and olive oils and mix with aroma essential oils: rosemary, lavender, rose, jasmine, sandalwood, lemon balm, etc. – 6 oz. oil & 6 drops essential oil. Web: aromatherapy.net or frontierherb.com

Massage – Self – Paul C. Bragg often said, "You can be your own best massage therapist, even if you have only one good hand." Near-miraculous improvements have been achieved by victims of accidents or strokes in bringing life back to afflicted parts of their own bodies by self-massage and even vibrators. Treatments can be day or night, almost continual. Self-massage also helps achieve relaxation at day's end. Families and friends can learn and exchange massages; it's a wonderful sharing experience. Remember, babies also love and thrive with daily massages – start from birth. Family pets also love the soothing, healing touch of massages. Web: amtamassage.org

Massage – Shiatsu – Japanese form of massage that applies pressure from the fingers, hands, elbows and even knees along the same points as acupuncture. Shiatsu has been used in Asia for centuries to relieve pain, common ills, muscle stress and to aid lymphatic circulation. Web: doubleclickd.com/Articles/shiatsu.html

126

Massage – Sports – An important support system for professional and amateur athletes. Sports massage: improves circulation and mobility to injured tissue, enables athletes to recover more rapidly from myofascial injury, reduces muscle soreness and chronic strain patterns. Soft tissues are freed of trigger points and adhesions, thus contributing to improvement of peak neuro-muscular functioning and athletic performance.

Massage – Swedish – One of the oldest and most widely used massage techniques. It's deep body massage that soothes, promotes circulation and is a great way to loosen and relax muscles before and after exercise. Web: massage-one.com/style.html

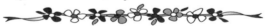

Author's Comment: My father and I have personally sampled many of these alternative therapies. It's estimated in the 21st century America's health care costs will leap over $2 trillion. It's more important than ever that we be responsible for our own health. This includes seeking holistic health practitioners who are dedicated to keeping us well by inspiring us to practice prevention! These Alternative Healing Therapies are also popular and getting results – color, aroma, music, biofeedback, Tai Chi, yoga, etc. Explore them and be open to improving your earthly temple for a healthy, happy, longer life. **Seek and find the best for your body, mind and soul.** – Patricia Bragg

A Personal Message to Our Students

It is our sincere desire that each one of our readers and students attain this precious super health and enjoy freedom from all nagging, tormenting human ailments.

After intelligent and careful study of this book, you now know that most human physical problems arise from a fermenting and decaying mass of toxins in the body. Many of these trouble spots are years old and are mainly concentrated in the intestines, colon and organs.

We have taught you that there is no special diet for any one special ailment! The Bragg Healthy Lifestyle promotes cleansing through the eating of more organic raw fruits and vegetables combined with regular fasting. It is only through progressive cleansing that the human "cesspool" can be banished! We have told you that you will go through healing crises from time to time. During these cleansing times you might have weakness and might become discouraged! This is the time you must have great strength and faith! It is during these crises, when you feel the worst, that you are doing the greatest amount of deep cleansing. This is why weaklings, cry-babies and people without will-power and intestinal fortitude fail to follow this perfect Bragg Heathy Lifestyle System of Cleansing and Rejuvenation! Please be strong!

Weaklings want a cure that requires no effort on their part. Mother Nature and your body do not work that way! The average unfortunate sick person thinks of the Lord as a kind and forgiving Father who will allow them to enter the Garden of Eden effortlessly and unpunished for any violation of His and Mother Nature's Laws.

You can create your own Garden of Eden anywhere you live, regardless of climate! All you have to do is to purify the body of its toxic poisons by living a healthy lifestyle. You can reach a stage of health and youthfulness that you never thought was possible! You can feel ageless where your chronological age actually stands still and pathological age will make you younger! When your body is free of deadly toxic material you will reach the physical, mental, emotional and spiritual state that will give you happiness every waking hour as it adds many more youthful, active, joyous years to your life.

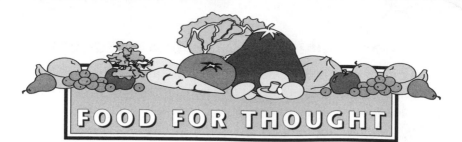

FOOD FOR THOUGHT

Flexibility goes a long way in helping you feel young. Joints and ligaments lose their elasticity if they aren't stretched, growing shorter and tighter. Tension also settles into unstretched muscles, further sapping energy, making one feel older, less energetic and less inclined to get up and move around. The good news is that you can improve your flexibility at any age because the body is remarkably resilient, as long as you pay attention to your own comfort levels and be consistent. Some rejuvenating stretches can be found in yoga, ballet, and basic sports stretches for all areas of the body. Remember to warm up before stretching by running in place, swinging your arms vigorously, to get the blood flowing. Don't bounce when you stretch. Don't hold your breath during stretches – gentle relaxed deep breathing is best. Be patient and don't push your body. While everyone can become more flexible, not everyone can be as limber as a dancer or gymnast. Challenge yourself, but don't push yourself further than you can realistically go. You'll be amazed at the results. And be consistent – it is the key to progress. – UC Berkeley Wellness Letter

Vitamin E is now known as the primary defender against damaging free radicals. Since stores of this nutrient decline with age, it is important to supplement your diet with vitamin E-rich foods such as wheat germ, nuts, green leafy vegetables and polyunsaturated vegetable oils. See page 106.

A recent study of nurses whose daily intake of 100 mgs and more of vitamin E had a 36% lower risk of heart attack and 23% lower risk of stroke.

Eating plenty of produce – fruits and vegetables – will slow down ageing. The ageing that goes on under the skin mantle and chronic age-associated diseases, including heart disease, cancer and degenerative brain diseases can be slowed down, and even reversed in some cases with a change in diet. Adding lots of fruits and vegetables and garlic, taking vitamin and mineral supplements, and avoiding saturated fat will add years to your life and increase your energy. Exercise is very important, also, in delaying ageing.
– Nanci Hellmich, USA Today

The use of antioxidant supplements and a diet high in antioxidant foods has been shown to reduce cancer and heart disease and increase life expectancy. Foods high in antioxidant vitamins include green vegetables, citrus fruits, nuts, whole grains, carrots, squash and cantaloupe. – U.S. News/Health Watch

A teacher for the day can be a guiding light for a lifetime!
Bragg books are silent health teachers – never tiring, ready night or day to help you help yourself to health! Our books are written with love and a deep desire to guide you to a healthy lifestyle. – Patricia Bragg

Earn Your Bragging Rights

Live The Bragg Healthy Lifestyle
To Attain Supreme Physical,
Mental, Emotional and Spiritual Health!

With your new awareness, understanding and sincere commitment of how to live The Bragg Healthy Lifestyle – you can now live a longer, healthier life to 120 years!

God bless you and your family and may He give you the strength, the courage and the patience to win your battle to re-enter the Healthy Garden of Eden while you are still living here on Earth with time to enjoy it all!

With Blessings of Health, Peace, Joy and Love,

Patricia and *Paul*

129

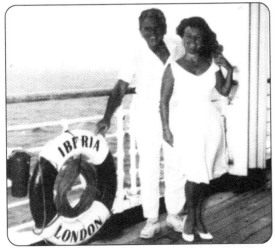

Health Crusaders Paul Bragg and daughter Patricia traveled the world spreading health, inspiring millions to renew and revitalize their health.

The Bragg books are written to inspire and guide you to health, fitness and longevity. Remember, the book you don't read won't help. So please read and reread the Bragg Books and live The Bragg Healthy Lifestyle!

I never suspected that I would have to learn how to live – that there were specific disciplines and ways of seeing the world that I had to master before I could awaken to a simple, healthy, happy, uncomplicated life. – Dan Millman

A truly good book teaches me better than to just read it, I must soon lay it down and commence living in its wisdom. What I began by reading, I must finish by acting! – Henry David Thoreau

PROMISE YOURSELF

• *Promise yourself to be so strong that nothing can disturb your peace of mind.*

• *To talk health, happiness and prosperity to every person you meet.*

• *To make your friends feel that they are special and appreciated.*

• *To look at the sunny side of everything and make your optimism come true.*

• *To think only of the best, to work only for the best and expect only the best.*

• *To be just as enthusiastic about the success of others as you are about your own.*

• *To forget the mistakes of the past and press on to the greater achievements of the future.*

• *To wear a cheerful countenance at all times and give every living creature you meet a smile.*

• *To give so much time to the improvement of yourself that you have no time to criticize others.*

• *To be too large for worry, too noble for anger, too strong for fear and too happy to permit the presence of trouble.*

– Christian D. Larson

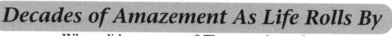

Decades of Amazement As Life Rolls By

130

Where did our years go? They went by so fast.
When we're young they seem to cra-a-wl,
With each decade, they fly past!

At 29 we're the center
At 30 we feel supreme
But 40 strikes terror;
Life's not what it seems.
By 50 we've reached maturity
At 60 we accept seniority.
When we're filled with

Excitement of creative living,
There's no room for depression and despair!

But at 65, wisdom that comes from experience
Then takes over and we learn
To accept ourselves as we are.
Each new day is a gift to be treasured,
Enabling us to go far!

Life is for the living
But it is through our sharing, loving and giving
That we reach for the Stars of
Joy, Peace and Possibilities for Eternity!

*– by Ruth Lubin, 88 years young & going strong,
who started writing poetry & sculpturing at 80!
PS: Ruth is a fan of the Bragg Healthy Lifestyle for over 58 years!*

Phytochemicals - Nature's Miracles Help Prevent Cancer

Make sure to get your daily dose of these naturally occurring, cancer-fighting biological substances that are abundant in tomatoes, onions, garlic, beans, legumes, soy beans, cabbage, cauliflower, broccoli, citrus fruits, etc. The champion – tomato, contains the highest count of phytochemicals!

Class	Food Sources	Action
PHYTOESTROGENS	Soy products, alfalfa sprouts, red clover sprouts, licorice root (not candy)	May block some cancers, & aids in menopausal symptoms
PHYTOSTEROLS	Plant oils, corn, soy, sesame, safflower, wheat, pumpkin	Blocks hormonal role in cancers, inhibits uptake of cholesterol from diet
SAPONINS	Yams, beets, beans, nuts, soybeans	May prevent cancer cells from multiplying
TERPENES	Carrots, yams, winter squash, sweet potatoes, apricots, cantaloupes	Antioxidants – protects DNA from free radical-induced damage
	Tomatoes and tomato-based products	Helps block UVA & UVB & may help protect against prostate cancers, etc.
	Citrus fruits (flavonoids)	Promotes protective enzymes; antiseptic
	Spinach, kale, beet & turnip greens	Protects eyes from macular degeneration
	Red chile peppers	Keeps carcinogens from binding to DNA
PHENOLS	Fennel, parsley, carrots, alfalfa	Prevents blood clotting & may have anticancer properties
	Citrus fruits, broccoli, cabbage, cucumbers, green peppers, tomatoes	Antioxidants – flavonoids block membrane receptor sites for certain hormones
	Grape seeds	Strong antioxidants; fights germs & bacteria, strengthens immune system, veins & capillaries
	Grapes, especially skins	Antioxidant, antimutagen; promotes detoxification. Acts as carcinogen inhibitors
	Yellow & green squash	Antihepatoxic, antitumor
SULFUR COMPOUNDS	Onions & garlic (fresh is best)	Promotes liver enzymes, inhibits cholesterol synthesis, reduces triglycerides, lowers blood pressure, improves immune response, fights infections, germs & parasites

❧❧❧❧❧ Morning Resolve ❧❧❧❧❧

I will this day live a simple, sincere and serene life. I will repel promptly every thought of impurity, discontent, anxiety, discouragement and self-seeking. I will cultivate cheerfulness, happiness, charity and the love of brotherhood; exercising economy in expenditure, generosity in giving, carefulness in conversation and diligence in appointed service. I pledge fidelity to every trust and a childlike faith in God. I will be faithful in my habits of prayer, study, work, physical exercise, deep breathing and good posture. I shall fast one 24 hour period each week, eat only natural foods and get sufficient sleep each night. I will make every effort to improve myself physically, mentally, emotionally and spiritually every day of my life.

Morning Prayer used by Patricia Bragg and her father, Paul C. Bragg

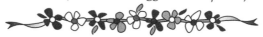

WE THANK THEE

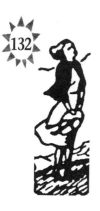

132

For flowers that bloom about our feet;
   For song of bird and hum of bee;
For all things fair we hear or see,
   Father in heaven we thank Thee!
For blue of stream and blue of sky;
   For pleasant shade of branches high;
For fragrant air and cooling breeze;
   For beauty of the blooming trees;
Father in heaven we thank Thee!
   For mother love and father care,
For brothers strong and sisters fair;
   For love at home and here each day;
For guidance lest we go astray,
   Father in heaven we thank Thee!
For this new morning with its light;
   For rest and shelter of the night;
For health and food, for love and friends;
   For every thing His goodness sends,
Father in heaven we thank Thee!
   – Ralph Waldo Emerson

MY DAILY HEALTH JOURNAL

Today is: /   /   /

I have said my morning resolve and am ready to practice
The Bragg Healthy Lifestyle today and every day.

Yesterday I went to bed at: Today I arose at:

Today I practiced the No-Heavy Breakfast or No-Breakfast Plan ☐ yes ☐ no
For Breakfast I drank   time:
For Breakfast I ate   time:
Supplements:

For Lunch I ate   time:
Supplements:

For Dinner I ate   time:
Supplements:

List Snacks – Kind and When:

I took part in these physical activities today:

Grade on a scale of 1 to 10 (10 being desired optimum health)
I rate my day for the following categories:
Previous Night's Sleep:
Elimination:
Energy Level:
Stress/Anxiety:
Physical Activity:
Health:
Peacefulness:
Self-Esteem:
Happiness:

General Comments and To Do List:

FROM THE AUTHORS

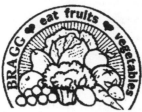

GO ORGANIC

This book was written for You! It can be your passport to a healthy, long, vital life. We in the Alternative Health Therapies join hands in one common objective – promoting a high standard of health for everyone. Healthy nutrition points the way – which is Mother Nature and God's Way. This book teaches you how to work with them, not against them. Health Doctors, therapists nurses, teachers and caregivers are becoming more dedicated than ever to keeping their patients healthy and fit. This book was written to speed the spread of this tremendous message of living a healthy lifestyle close to Mother Nature and God.

Statements in this book are scientific health findings, known facts of physiology and biological therapeutics. Paul C. Bragg practiced the natural methods of living for over 80 years with highly beneficial results, knowing that they were safe and of great value. His daughter Patricia Bragg worked with him and continues to carry on the Bragg Health Crusades.

Paul C. Bragg and daughter Patricia express their opinions solely as Public Health Educators and Health Crusaders. They offer no cure for disease. Only the body has the ability to cure a person. Experts may disagree with some of the statements made in this book. However, such statements are considered to be factual, based on the long-time health experience of pioneers Paul C. Bragg and Patricia Bragg. If you suspect you have a medical problem, please seek alternative health professionals to help you make the healthiest, wisest and best-informed choices.

Oxygen is the main nutrient of the body. When we improve our oxygen intake, we enhance our immune system and the body's ability to detoxify and stay healthy. – Dr. Michael Schachter, Columbia University

---

Jesus said, "Thy faith hath made thee whole, now go and sin no more." That includes your dietetic sins! He Himself, through fasting and prayer, was able to heal the sick and cure all manner of diseases.

To maintain good health, normal weight and increase the good life of radiant health, joy and happiness, the body must be exercised properly (stretching, walking, jogging, running, biking, swimming, deep breathing, good posture, etc.) and nourished wisely with natural foods. – Paul C. Bragg

Index

A

Abdomen, 79, 101, 110
Abscesses, 26, 96
Acerola, 96, 128
Aches, 2-4, 6-7, 15, 18, 37, 41, 45, 65
  ear-, 26
  head-, 4, 6, 26, 34, 50, 69
  muscle, 125, 126
Acid, 6, 18, 69
  tannic, 70
  toxic, 18, 76
  uric, 18, 51, 88, 94
Acupressure, 123
Acupuncture, 123
Adjustments, 38, 121-122
Age, 2, 12, 19, 22, 28, 31, 33, 45,
  47, 60, 62, 67, 81, 95, 107, 127
  biological, 12
  chronological, 12, 127
  pathological, 127
Ageing, 7-8, 12, 18-19, 47, 109
Agelessness, 13, 15-16, 31-33, 47, 127
Air, 29, 46, 78, 83-84, 90, 92
Air purifiers, 21
Alcohol, 7, 9, 22, 25, 32,
  43, 54, 96, 104
Alexander Technique, 123
Alfalfa, 70, 96, 108
Allergies, food, 100, 112
Aloe gel drink, 66
Animals, 18-19, 28, 51, 53, 57
Ankles, swollen, 80, 104,
Antioxidents, 120-121, 128
Anxiety, 6, 72, 77
Apple Cider Vinegar - ACV, 25, 28,
  48-49, 62, 66-67, 86, 105,
  108-109, 114, 116, 124
ACV cocktail, 48, 108-109, 114
Apples, 17, 29, 37, 57, 66, 79, 82,
  85, 99, 108, 114
Apricots, 17, 62, 99, 113-114
Aroma Therapy, 125
Arteries, 22, 45, 52, 108
  hardening of, 11-13, 15, 52

Arthritis, 9, 28, 108
Aspartame, 12, 19, 23, 42, 67, 89, 120
Assimilation, 25, 40
Asthma, 19, 24, 88
Athletes, 48, 80, 90, 120
Avocado, 49, 115, 123-124

B

Babies, 27, 29, 123
Back, 30, 35, 79, 83, 90,
Bacteria, 83, 86, 91, 108, 116
Bathing
  air, 78
  sun, 75-78
  tub, 124
Beano, digestive aid, 68
Beans, 17-18, 24, 28, 46, 50-52,
  61, 66-67, 92, 94, 103, 113, 117
  dried, 51-52
Biking, 81, 130
Biochemistry, human laws of, 22
Biofeedback, 91, 124
Bioflavonoids, 96
Blindness, 9, 15
Blood, 7, 11, 40, 60, 78, 80, 91,
  97, 101, 116, 118, 120, 126
  chemistry values, 121
  pressure, 45, 51, 72, 93, 100,
  115, 120, 124
  sugar, 40-41
Bloodstream, 4, 7, 9, 15, 23, 40, 52,
  61, 71, 92 96-97, 107, 120
Bones, 2, 6, 15, 19, 28, 32, 77, 108, 118
Boron, 28
Bowels, 4, 50, 101-104
Bragg, Dr. Paul C., 10, 27, 35, 42,
  47, 59, 62, 64, 71, 84, 99-100, 112,
  116, 120, 123, 128-129
Bragg Liquid Aminos, 25, 48, 54, 98,
  114-115
Brain, 7, 13, 117, 126
Breads, 12, 19, 23, 29, 46, 53, 60,
  63-64, 66-67, 95, 113-114, 117

"I conceive that a knowledge of books is the basis on which all other knowledge rests." – President George Washington

136

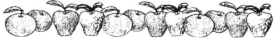

If families could be induced to substitute the healthy organic apple, sound, ripe and luscious, in place of white sugar, white flour pies, cakes, candies and other sweets with which children are too often stuffed, doctors' bills would diminish sufficiently enough in a single year to lay up a stock of this delicious fruit for a season's use.

137

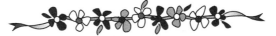

Simplify – Simplify – Simplify – Your Life!

*Streamline and unclutter your home and closets, your business
and office, your professional and personal life of all unnecessary
baggage in this overly modern, yet hectic world of today!
Live simply and stay close to Mother Nature and God! – Patricia Bragg*

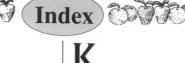
H

I

J

K

L

M

138

Fruit bears the closest relation to light. The sun pours a continuous flood of light into the fruits, and they furnish the best potion of food a human being requires for the mind and body – Louisa May Alcott

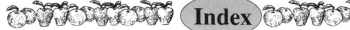

139

Important Health Facts!

Scientists at the Department of Agriculture's Human Nutrition Research Center on Ageing in Boston report that daily requirements for vitamins B-6, B-12, C, D and E escalate with age, along with the need for calcium, beta-carotene and folic acid. Play it safe – be sure to take multi-vitamin and mineral supplements.

We are recharged and blessed by each one of you reading our healthy teaching, living, loving words – thank you! – Patricia Bragg

We must always change, renew, rejuvenate; otherwise, we harden.– Goethe

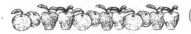 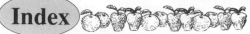

Index

Those who do good of their own accord shall be rewarded, but to fast is better for you, if you knew it. – Mohammed, 500-600 A.D.

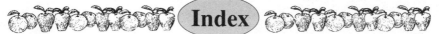

Index

141

**HAVE AN APPLE
HEALTHY LIFE!**

Old age is not a time of life. It is a condition of the body. It is not time that ages the body, it is abuse that does! – Herbert M. Shelton

Children are very responsive to healthy lifestyle changes, and those start with providing the right foods (fruits, vegetables, whole grains and reasonable amounts of other healthful snacks), encouraging regular exercise and activity and limiting television watching!
– Susan K. Rhodes, Ph.D., Medical University of South Carolina

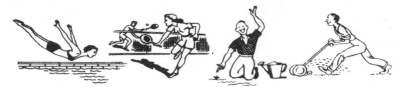

The Bragg Healthy Lifestyle
For a Lifetime of Super Health

In a broad sense, "The Bragg Healthy Lifestyle for the Total Person" is a combination of physical, mental, emotional, social and spiritual components. The ability of the individual to function effectively in his environment depends on how smoothly these components function as a whole. Of all the qualities that comprise an integrated personality, a totally healthy, fit body is one of the most desirable . . . so start today for achieving your health goals!

A person may be said to be totally physically fit if he functions as a total personality with efficiency and without pain or discomfort of any kind. This is to have a Painless, Tireless, Ageless body, possessing sufficient muscular strength and endurance to maintain a healthy posture and successfully carry on the duties imposed by life and the environment, to meet emergencies satisfactorily and have enough energy for recreation and social obligations after the "work day" has ended. It is to meet the requirements of his environment through possessing the resilience to recover rapidly from fatigue, tension, stress and strain of daily living without the aid of stimulants, drugs or alcohol, and enjoy natural recharging sleep at night and awaken fit and alert in the morning for the challenges of the new fresh day ahead.

Keeping the body totally healthy and fit is not a job for the uninformed or the careless person. It requires an understanding of the body and of a healthy lifestyle and then following it for a long, happy lifetime of health! The result of "The Bragg Healthy Lifestyle" is to wake up the possibilities within you, rejuvenate your body, mind and soul to total balanced health. It's within your reach, so don't procrastinate, start today! Our hearts go out to touch your heart with nourishing, caring love for your total health!

Patricia Bragg and Paul C. Bragg

Dear friend, I wish above all things that thou may prosper and be in health even as the soul prospers. – 3 John 2

Send for Free Health Bulletins

Patricia Bragg wants to keep in touch with you, your relatives and friends about the latest Health, Nutrition, Exercise and Longevity Discoveries. Please enclose two stamps for each USA name listed. Foreign listings send postal reply coupons.

With Blessings of Health and Thanks,

Please print or type addresses clearly . . .

Patricia

BRAGG HEALTH CRUSADES, Box 7, Santa Barbara, CA 93102
You can help too!
Keep the Bragg Health Crusades "crusading" with your tax-deductible gifts.

Name
_____

Address _____ Apt. No.

City _____ State _____ Zip _____

Phone ( ) E-mail

- -

Name
_____

Address _____ Apt. No.

City _____ State _____ Zip _____

Phone ( ) E-mail

- -

Name
_____

Address _____ Apt. No.

City _____ State _____ Zip _____

Phone ( ) E-mail

Dear Patricia, Yes! I want to be a Bragg Health Crusader . . .

Enclosed is my gift of ☐ $5 ☐ $20 ☐ $50 ☐ $100 ☐ $_____

Your gifts to the Bragg Health Crusades are tax-deductible in the USA.

Name
_____

Address _____ Apt. No.

City _____ State _____ Zip _____

Phone ( ) E-mail

Bragg Health Crusades spreading health worldwide over 87 years

Bragg Organic Raw Apple Cider Vinegar
With the Mother . . . Nature's Delicious, Healthy Miracle

**HAVE AN
APPLE
HEALTHY
LIFE!**

IF? Your Health Store
doesn't carry Bragg Books,
Bragg Aminos
and Bragg Vinegar
Ask them to contact their
Health Distributor to
stock them! Or call Bragg
at 800-446-1990

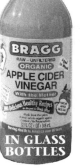

IN GLASS
BOTTLES

INTERNAL BENEFITS:
- Rich Miracle Enzymes & Potassium
- Natural Antibiotic & Germ Fighter
- Helps Control & Normalize Weight
- Improves Digestion & Assimilation
- Helps Fight Arthritis & Stiffness
- Relieves Sore & Dry Throat
- Helps Remove Toxins & Sludge

EXTERNAL BENEFITS:
- Helps Promote Youthful, Healthy Body
- Helps Promote & Maintain Healthy Skin
- Soothes Sunburn, Shingles & Bites
- Helps Prevent Dandruff & Itchy Scalp
- Soothes, Aching Joints & Muscles

BRAGG ORGANIC APPLE CIDER VINEGAR

SIZE	PRICE	USA SHIPPING & HANDLING	AMT	$ TOTAL
16 oz.	$ 2.19 each	Please add $4 for 1st bottle and $1.50 each additional bottle		.
16 oz	$ 21.00 Case/12	S/H Cost by Time Zone: CA $8. PST/MST $9. CST $13. EST $15.		.
32 oz.	$ 3.79 each	Please add $5 for 1st bottle and $2.00 each additional bottle.		.
32 oz.	$ 40.00 Case/12	S/H Cost by Time Zone: CA $11. PST/MST $14. CST $21. EST $25.		.
1 gal.	$ 12.98 each	S/H 1st bottle: CA $6. PST/MST $7. CST $8. EST $9. – $5. @ add'l. bottle.		.
1 gal.	$ 47.00 Case/4	S/H Cost by Time Zone: CA $11. PST/MST $15. CST $23. EST $27.		.

Bragg Vinegar is a food and not taxable

Foreign orders, please inquire on postage

Please Specify: ☐ Check ☐ Money Order ☐ Cash

Charge To: ☐ Visa ☐ MasterCard ☐ Discover

Total Vinegar $	.
Shipping & Handling	.
Total Enclosed $ (USA Funds Only)	.

Credit Card
Number: _ _ _ _ _ _ _ _ _ _ _ _ _ _ _ _   Card Expires: Month | Year

MasterCard   *VISA*   DISCOVER   **Signature:** _____

CREDIT CARD ORDERS ONLY
CALL: **(800) 446-1990**
FAX: **(805) 968-1001**
EMAIL: **bragg@bragg.com**

Business office calls (805) 968-1020. We accept MasterCard
Discover or VISA phone orders. Please prepare your order using this
order form. It will speed your call and serve as your order record.
Hours: 9 am to 4 pm Pacific Time, Monday thru Thursday.
Visit our Web Site: http://www.bragg.com & e-mail: bragg@bragg.com

Mail to: **HEALTH SCIENCE, Box 7, Santa Barbara, CA 93102 USA**

Please Print or Type – Be sure to give street & house number to facilitate delivery.

V-BOF-904

Name
_____

Address _____ Apt. No. _____

City _____ State _____ Zip _____

Phone ( ) _____ ● E-mail _____

Bragg Organic, Raw Apple Cider Vinegar
Available Health Stores - Nationwide

BRAGG "HOW-TO, SELF-HEALTH" BOOKS
Authored by America's First Family of Health
Live Longer – Healthier – Stronger Self-Improvement Library

Qty.	Bragg Book Titles ORDER FORM Health Science ISBN 0-87790	Price	$ Total
___	Apple Cider Vinegar — Miracle Health System (6 million in print)	6.95	.
___	The Bragg Healthy Lifestyle - Vital Living to 120 (formerly Toxicless Diet)	7.95	.
___	Super Power Breathing for Super Energy and High Health	7.95	.
___	Miracle of Fasting (Bragg Bible of Health for physical rejuvenation & longevity)	8.95	.
___	Water – The Shocking Truth (learn safest water to drink & why)	7.95	.
___	Nature's Healing System to Improve Eyesight	7.95	.
___	Bragg's Complete Gourmet Health Recipes for Super Health – 448 pages	8.95	.
___	Build Powerful Nerve Force (reduce stress, fear, anger, worry)	7.95	.
___	Keep Your Heart & Cardiovascular System Healthy & Fit at Any Age	7.95	.
___	Nature's Way to Reduce (lose 10 pounds in 10 days)	6.95	.
___	Hair and Your Health, Nature's Way to Beautiful Hair (easy-to-do method)	7.95	.
___	Healthy, Strong Feet – "Best Complete Foot Program" – Dr. Scholl	7.95	.

BRAGG LECTURE TAPES, VIDEO, CD ROM & CDs

Qty.		Price	$ Total
___	Patricia & Paul Bragg – Famous Health Lectures (70 min. Cassette Tape)	5.95	.
___	Patricia & Paul Bragg – Famous Health Lectures (70 min. CD)	11.95	.
___	Bragg Variety – Now on VHS: Patricia & Paul's Lectures, Exercises, Recipes, etc. ..	7.95	.
___	Bragg Collection – Interactive CD Rom: Lectures, Exercises, Recipes & more ..	11.95	.

Total Items   Prices subject to change without notice.

TOTAL ITEMS	$.
CA residents add sales tax	.
Shipping & Handling	.
TOTAL ENCLOSED (USA Funds Only)	$.

USA Shipping Please add $3.50 for first book, tape CD, etc.
Add $1.00 for each additional item
USA retail book, tape & CD orders over $35 add $5 only
Canada & Foreign orders add $4 first item $2 each additional

Please Specify:
Charge To: ☐ Visa ☐ Master Card ☐ Discover ☐ Check ☐ Cash ☐ Money Order   Month | Year

Credit Card #: _ _ _ _ _ _ _ _ _ _ _ _ _ _ _ _   Card Expires: ___|___

MasterCard   VISA   DISCOVER   **Signature:** _____

FREE GIFT– 70 minutes with Patricia & Paul Bragg!
with orders of $30 or more receive a Free CD or casette tape.

✓ Check one: ☐ CD ☐ Casette Tape

CREDIT CARD ORDERS ONLY
CALL: **(800) 446-1990**
FAX: (805) 968-1001
EMAIL: bragg@bragg.com

Business office calls (805) 968-1020. We accept MasterCard Discover or VISA phone orders. Please prepare your order using this order form. It will speed your call and serve as your order record. Hours: 9 am to 4 pm Pacific Time, Monday thru Thursday.
Visit our Web Site: http://www.bragg.com & e-mail: bragg@bragg.com

Mail to: **HEALTH SCIENCE, Box 7, Santa Barbara, CA 93102 USA**

Please Print or Type – Be sure to give street & house number to facilitate delivery.   B-BOF-904

Name _____

Address _____   Apt. No. _____

City _____   State _____   Zip _____

Phone ( ) _____   E-mail _____

Bragg Books are available most Health & Book Stores – Nationwide

BRAGG "HOW-TO, SELF-HEALTH" BOOKS

Authored by America's First Family of Health
Live Longer – Healthier – Stronger Self-Improvement Library

Qty.	Bragg Book Titles ORDER FORM Health Science ISBN 0-87790	Price	$ Total
_____	**Apple Cider Vinegar — Miracle Health System** (6 million in print)	6.95	_____ .
_____	**The Bragg Healthy Lifestyle - Vital Living to 120** (formerly Toxicless Diet)	7.95	_____ .
_____	**Super Power Breathing for Super Energy and High Health**	7.95	_____ .
_____	**Miracle of Fasting** (Bragg Bible of Health for physical rejuvenation & longevity)	8.95	_____ .
_____	**Water – The Shocking Truth** (learn safest water to drink & why)	7.95	_____ .
_____	**Nature's Healing System to Improve Eyesight**	7.95	_____ .
_____	**Bragg's Complete Gourmet Health Recipes** for Super Health – 448 pages	8.95	_____ .
_____	**Build Powerful Nerve Force** (reduce stress, fear, anger, worry)	7.95	_____ .
_____	**Keep Your Heart & Cardiovascular System Healthy & Fit** at Any Age	7.95	_____ .
_____	**Nature's Way to Reduce** (lose 10 pounds in 10 days)	6.95	_____ .
_____	**Hair and Your Health**, Nature's Way to Beautiful Hair (easy-to-do method)	7.95	_____ .
_____	**Healthy, Strong Feet** – "Best Complete Foot Program" – Dr. Scholl	7.95	_____ .

BRAGG LECTURE TAPES, VIDEO, CD ROM & CDs

_____	**Patricia & Paul Bragg** – Famous Health Lectures (70 min. **Cassette Tape**)	5.95	_____ .
_____	**Patricia & Paul Bragg** – Famous Health Lectures (70 min. **CD**)	11.95	_____ .
_____	**Bragg Variety** – Now on **VHS**: Patricia & Paul's Lectures, Exercises, Recipes, etc. ..	7.95	_____ .
_____	**Bragg Collection** – Interactive **CD Rom**: Lectures, Exercises, Recipes & more ..	11.95	_____ .

Total Items Prices subject to change without notice.	**TOTAL ITEMS** $.

USA Shipping ➤ Please add $3.50 for first book, tape CD, etc.
Add $1.00 for each additional item

	CA residents add sales tax	.
USA retail book, tape & CD orders over $35 add $5 only	**Shipping & Handling**	.
Canada & Foreign orders add $4 first item $2 each additional	**TOTAL ENCLOSED** $ (USA Funds Only)	.

Please Specify:
Charge To: ☐ Visa ☐ Master Card ☐ Discover ☐ Check ☐ Cash ☐ Money Order   Month | Year

Credit Card **#**: _ _ _ _ _ _ _ _ _ _ _ _ _ _ _ _   Card Expires: _____

MasterCard   VISA   DISCOVER   **Signature:** _____

FREE GIFT– 70 minutes with Patricia & Paul Bragg!
with orders of $30 or more receive a Free CD or casette tape.
✓ Check one: ☐ CD ☐ Casette Tape

CREDIT CARD ORDERS ONLY	**Business office calls (805) 968-1020.** We accept MasterCard
CALL: **(800) 446-1990**	Discover or VISA phone orders. Please prepare your order using this
FAX: **(805) 968-1001**	order form. It will speed your call and serve as your order record.
EMAIL: **bragg@bragg.com**	Hours: 9 am to 4 pm Pacific Time, Monday thru Thursday. Visit our Web Site: http://www.bragg.com & e-mail: bragg@bragg.com

Mail to: **HEALTH SCIENCE, Box 7, Santa Barbara, CA 93102 USA**

Please Print or Type – Be sure to give street & house number to facilitate delivery.   B-BOF-904

•
Name

•   •
Address   Apt. No.

•
City   State   Zip

Phone (   )   ● E-mail

BRAGG ALL NATURAL LIQUID AMINOS

Healthy, Delicious Seasoning Alternative to Tamari & Soy Sauce

BRAGG LIQUID AMINOS – Nutrition you need...taste you will love...a family favorite for over 87 years. A delicious source of nutritious life-renewing protein from soy beans only. Add to or spray over casseroles, soups, sauces, gravies, potatoes, popcorn, and vegetables. An ideal "pick-me-up" broth at work, home or the gym. Gourmet health replacement for Tamari and Soy Sauce. Start today and add more Amino Acids to your daily diet for healthy living – the easy BRAGG LIQUID AMINOS Way!

SPRAY or DASH brings NEW TASTE DELIGHTS! PROVEN & ENJOYED BY MILLIONS.

Now in Handy 6 oz Spray Bottle

Spray or Dash of Bragg Aminos Brings New Taste Delights to Season:

- Salads
- Dressings
- Soups
- Veggies
- Tofu
- Rice/Beans
- Tempeh
- Stir-frys
- Wok foods
- Gravies
- Sauces
- Meats
- Poultry
- Fish
- Popcorn
- Casseroles & Potatoes
- Macrobiotics

Pure Soy Beans and Pure Water Only

- No Added Sodium
- No Coloring Agents
- No Preservatives
- Not Fermented
- No Chemicals
- No Additives

BRAGG LIQUID AMINOS

SIZE	PRICE	USA SHIPPING & HANDLING	AMT	$ TOTAL
6 oz.	$ 2.98 each	Please add $3. for 1st 3 bottles – $1.25 each additional bottle.		
6 oz.	$ 65.00 Case/24	S/H Cost by Time Zone: CA $6. PST/MST $8. CST $10. EST $12.		
16 oz.	$ 3.95 each	Please add $3. for 1st bottle – $1.25 each additional bottle.		
16 oz.	$ 42.00 Case/12	S/H Cost by Time Zone: CA $7. PST/MST $8. CST $11. EST $13.		
32 oz.	$ 6.45 each	Please add $4. for 1st bottle – $1.50 each additional bottle.		
32 oz.	$ 70.00 Case/12	S/H Cost by Time Zone: CA $9. PST/MST $12. CST $17. EST $20.		
1 gal.	$ 23.50 each	S/H 1st bottle: CA $6. PST/MST $7. CST $8. EST $9. – $5. @ add'l. bottle.		
1 gal.	$ 89.00 Case/4	S/H Cost by Time Zone: CA $12. PST/MST $15. CST $22. EST $27.		

Bragg Liquid Aminos is a food and not taxable

Foreign orders, please inquire on postage

Please Specify: ☐ Check ☐ Money Order ☐ Cash

Charge To: ☐ Visa ☐ MasterCard ☐ Discover

Credit Card Number:

Total Aminos $	
Shipping & Handling	
Total Enclosed $ (USA Funds Only)	

Card Expires: _____ Month _____ Year

MasterCard VISA DISCOVER **Signature:** _____

CREDIT CARD ORDERS ONLY
CALL: **(800) 446-1990**
FAX: **(805) 968-1001**
EMAIL: **bragg@bragg.com**

Business office calls (805) 968-1020. We accept MasterCard Discover or VISA phone orders. Please prepare your order using this order form. It will speed your call and serve as your order record. Hours: 9 am to 4 pm Pacific Time, Monday thru Thursday.
Visit our Web Site: http://www.bragg.com & e-mail: bragg@bragg.com

Mail to: HEALTH SCIENCE, Box 7, Santa Barbara, CA 93102 USA

Please Print or Type – Be sure to give street & house number to facilitate delivery.

A-BOF-904

Name

Address / Apt. No.

City / State / Zip

Phone ( ) / E-mail

Bragg Aminos – Taste You Love, Nutrition You Need!
Available Health Stores - Nationwide

BRAGG "HOW-TO, SELF-HEALTH" BOOKS

Authored by America's First Family of Health
Live Longer – Healthier – Stronger Self-Improvement Library

Qty.	Bragg Book Titles ORDER FORM Health Science ISBN 0-87790	Price	$ Total
____	**Apple Cider Vinegar — Miracle Health System** (6 million in print)	6.95	____
____	**The Bragg Healthy Lifestyle - Vital Living to 120** (formerly Toxicless Diet)	7.95	____
____	**Super Power Breathing for Super Energy and High Health**	7.95	____
____	**Miracle of Fasting** (Bragg Bible of Health for physical rejuvenation & longevity)	8.95	____
____	**Water – The Shocking Truth** (learn safest water to drink & why)	7.95	____
____	**Nature's Healing System to Improve Eyesight**	7.95	____
____	**Bragg's Complete Gourmet Health Recipes** for Super Health – 448 pages	8.95	____
____	**Build Powerful Nerve Force** (reduce stress, fear, anger, worry)	7.95	____
____	**Keep Your Heart & Cardiovascular System Healthy & Fit** at Any Age	7.95	____
____	**Nature's Way to Reduce** (lose 10 pounds in 10 days)	6.95	____
____	**Hair and Your Health**, Nature's Way to Beautiful Hair (easy-to-do method)	7.95	____
____	**Healthy, Strong Feet** – "Best Complete Foot Program" – Dr. Scholl	7.95	____

BRAGG LECTURE TAPES, VIDEO, CD ROM & CDs

Qty.		Price	$ Total
____	**Patricia & Paul Bragg** – Famous Health Lectures (70 min. **Cassette Tape**)	5.95	____
____	**Patricia & Paul Bragg** – Famous Health Lectures (70 min. **CD**)	11.95	____
____	**Bragg Variety** – Now on **VHS**: Patricia & Paul's Lectures, Exercises, Recipes, etc. ..	7.95	____
____	**Bragg Collection** – Interactive **CD Rom**: Lectures, Exercises, Recipes & more ..	11.95	____

Total Items [____] Prices subject to change without notice.

TOTAL ITEMS	$ ____
CA residents add sales tax	____
Shipping & Handling	____
TOTAL ENCLOSED (USA Funds Only)	$ ____

USA Shipping > Please add $3.50 for first book, tape CD, etc.
Add $1.00 for each additional item
USA retail book, tape & CD orders over $35 add $5 only
Canada & Foreign orders add $4 first item $2 each additional

Please Specify:
Charge To: ☐ Visa ☐ Master Card ☐ Discover ☐ Check ☐ Cash ☐ Money Order   Month   Year

Credit Card **#:** ___ ___ ___ ___ — ___ ___ ___ ___ — ___ ___ ___ ___ — ___ ___ ___ ___   Card Expires: ____ | ____

MasterCard VISA DISCOVER   **Signature:** _____

FREE GIFT– 70 minutes with Patricia & Paul Bragg!
with orders of $30 or more receive a Free CD or casette tape.

✓ Check one: ☐ CD ☐ Casette Tape

CREDIT CARD ORDERS ONLY
CALL: **(800) 446-1990**
FAX: **(805) 968-1001**
EMAIL: **bragg@bragg.com**

Business office calls (805) 968-1020. We accept MasterCard Discover or VISA phone orders. Please prepare your order using this order form. It will speed your call and serve as your order record. Hours: 9 am to 4 pm Pacific Time, Monday thru Thursday.
Visit our Web Site: http://www.bragg.com & e-mail: bragg@bragg.com

Mail to: **HEALTH SCIENCE, Box 7, Santa Barbara, CA 93102 USA**

Please Print or Type – Be sure to give street & house number to facilitate delivery.   B-BOF-904

● _____
Name

● _____ ● _____
Address   Apt. No.

● _____
City   State   Zip

Phone (___) _____   ● E-mail _____

Bragg Books are available most Health & Book Stores – Nationwide

Send for Free Health Bulletins

Patricia Bragg wants to keep in touch with you, your relatives and friends about the latest Health, Nutrition, Exercise and Longevity Discoveries. Please enclose two stamps for each USA name listed. Foreign listings send postal reply coupons.

With Blessings of Health and Thanks,

Patricia

Please print or type addresses clearly . . .

BRAGG HEALTH CRUSADES, Box 7, Santa Barbara, CA 93102
You can help too!
Keep the Bragg Health Crusades "crusading" with your tax-deductible gifts.

Name _____

Address _____ Apt. No. ____

City _____ State _____ Zip _____

Phone (_____) _____ ● E-mail _____

Name _____

Address _____ Apt. No. ____

City _____ State _____ Zip _____

Phone (_____) _____ ● E-mail _____

Name _____

Address _____ Apt. No. ____

City _____ State _____ Zip _____

Phone (_____) _____ ● E-mail _____

Dear Patricia, Yes! I want to be a Bragg Health Crusader . . .
Enclosed is my gift of ☐ $5 ☐ $20 ☐ $50 ☐ $100 ☐ $_____
Your gifts to the Bragg Health Crusades are tax-deductible in the USA.

Name _____

Address _____ Apt. No. ____

City _____ State _____ Zip _____

Phone (_____) _____ ● E-mail _____

Bragg Health Crusades spreading health worldwide over 87 years

PAUL C. BRAGG N.D., Ph.D.

Life Extension Specialist • World Health Crusader
Lecturer and Advisor to Olympic Athletes, Royalty and Stars
Originator of Health Food Stores – Now Worldwide

For almost a Century, Living Proof that his
"Health and Fitness Way of Life" Works Wonders!

Paul C. Bragg is the Father of the Health Movement in America. This dynamic Crusader for worldwide health and fitness is responsible for more *firsts* in the history of the Health Movement than any other individual.

Bragg's amazing pioneering achievements the world now enjoys:

- Bragg originated, named and opened the first Health Food Store in America.
- Bragg Health Crusades pioneered the first Health Lectures across America. Bragg inspired followers to open health stores across America and also worldwide.
- Bragg introduced pineapple juice and tomato juice to the American public.
- He was the first to introduce and distribute honey nationwide.
- He introduced Juice Therapy in America by importing the first hand-juicers.
- Bragg pioneered Radio Health Programs from Hollywood three times daily.
- Paul and Patricia pioneered a Health TV show from Hollywood to spread *Health and Happiness* . . . the name of the show! It included exercises, health recipes, visual demonstrations and guest appearances by famous, health-minded people.
- He opened the first health restaurants and the first health spas in America.
- He created the first health foods and products and made them available nationwide: herb teas, health beverages, seven-grain cereals and crackers, health cosmetics, health candies, calcium, vitamins and mineral supplements, wheat germ, digestive enzymes from papaya, herbs and kelp seasonings, and amino acids from soy beans. Bragg inspired others to follow (Schiff, Shaklee, Twin Labs, Herbalife, etc.) and now thousands of health items are available worldwide.

Crippled by TB as a teenager, Bragg developed his own eating, breathing and exercising program to rebuild his body into an ageless, tireless, pain-free citadel of glowing, radiant, super health. He excelled in running, swimming, biking, progressive weight training and mountain climbing. He made an early pledge to God, in return for his renewed health, to spend the rest of his life showing others the road to health. He honored his pledge! Paul Bragg's health pioneering made a difference worldwide.

A legend and beloved counselor to millions, Bragg was the inspiration and personal health and fitness advisor to top Olympic Stars from 4-time swimming Gold Medalist Murray Rose to 3-time track Gold Medalist Betty Cuthbert of Australia, his relative (pole-vaulting Gold Medalist), Don Bragg and countless others. Jack LaLanne, the original TV Fitness King , says, *"Bragg saved my life at age 15 when I attended the Bragg Crusade in Oakland, California."* From the earliest days, Bragg advised the greatest Hollywood Stars and giants of American Business. J. C. Penney, Del E. Webb, Dr. Scholl and Conrad Hilton are just a few who he inspired to long, successful, healthy, active lives!

Dr. Bragg changed the lives of millions worldwide in all walks of life with the Bragg Health Crusades, Books, Tapes, Radio and TV appearances.

BRAGG HEALTH CRUSADES, Box 7, SANTA BARBARA, CA 93102 USA

PATRICIA BRAGG N.D., Ph.D.

Angel of Health and Healing

Author, Lecturer, Nutritionist, Health Educator & Fitness Advisor to World Leaders, Hollywood Stars, Singers, Dancers, Athletes, etc.

Daughter of the world renowned health authority, Paul C. Bragg, Patricia has won international fame on her own in this field. She conducts Health and Fitness Seminars for Women's, Men's, Youth and Church Groups throughout the world . . . and promotes Bragg "How-To, Self-Health" Books in Lectures, on Radio and Television Talk Shows throughout the world. Consultants to Presidents and Royalty, to the Stars of Stage, Screen and TV and to Champion Athletes, Patricia and her father are Co-Authors of the Bragg Health Library of Instructive, Inspiring Books that promote a longer, vital, healthier lifestyle.

Patricia herself is the symbol of health, perpetual youth and super energy. She is a live sparkling example of her and her father's healthy lifestyle precepts. She loves sharing this message with people worldwide. From an early childhood desire to be a missionary, Patricia fulfilled her dream by becoming a global missionary of health, as her father before her!

A fifth-generation Californian on her mother's side, Patricia was reared by The Bragg Natural Health Method from infancy. In school, she not only excelled in athletics, but also won honors for her studies and her counseling. She is an accomplished musician and dancer . . . as well as tennis player and mountain climber . . . and the youngest woman ever to be granted a U.S. Patent. Patricia is a popular gifted Health Teacher and a dynamic, in-demand Talk Show Guest where she spreads with a devoted passion the simple, easy-to-follow Bragg Healthy Lifestyle for everyone.

Man's body is his vehicle through life, his earthly temple . . . and the Creator wants us filled with joy & health for a long fruitful life. The Bragg Crusades of Health and Fitness (3 John 2) have carried her around the world over 13 times, spreading health – physically, mentally, emotionally and spiritually. Health is our birthright and Patricia teaches how simple it is to prevent the destruction of health from man-made unhealthy living habits.

Patricia's been a Health Consultant to American Presidents and British Royalty, to Betty Cuthbert, Australia's "Golden Girl," who holds 16 world records and four Olympic gold medals in women's track and to New Zealand's Olympic Track and Triathlete Star, Allison Roe. Among those who come to her for advice are some of Hollywood's top Stars from Clint Eastwood to the ever-youthful singing group, The Beach Boys and their families, Singing Stars of the Metropolitan Opera and top Ballet Stars. Patricia's message is of world-wide appeal to people of all ages, nationalities and walks-of-life. Those who follow The Bragg Healthy Lifestyle and attend the Bragg Crusades worldwide are living testimonials . . . like ageless, super athlete, Jack LaLanne, who at age 15 went from sickness to Total Health!

Patricia inspires people worldwide to Renew, Rejuvenate and Revitalize their life with *The Bragg Healthy Lifestyle* Books and Crusades. Millions have benefitted from these life-changing events with a longer, healthier and happier life! She loves to share with your community, organization, church groups, etc. Also, she is a perfect radio and TV talk show guest to spread the message of healthy lifestyle living. See Patricia on the web: bragg.com.

For Radio interview requests and info write or call (805) 968-1020
BRAGG HEALTH CRUSADES, BOX 7, SANTA BARBARA, CA 93102, USA